THE REALITY OF DYSLEXIA

Other titles in the Cassell Education series:

The Reality of Dyslexia

John Osmond

With a Foreword by T. R. Miles

CASSELL

in association with Channel Four Television

This book is for
Tomos Rhys

Cassell
Wellington House
125 Strand
London WC2R 0BB

215 Park Avenue South
New York
NY 10003

© John Osmond 1993

First published 1993
Reprinted 1994, 1996

British Library Cataloguing-in-Publication Data
A catalogue record for this book is available from the British Library

ISBN: 0-304-32762-X (hardback)
        0-304-32763-8 (paperback)

Typeset by Colset Private Limited, Singapore
Printed and bound in Great Britain by
Biddles Limited, Guildford and King's Lynn

Contents

Foreword

by Professor T. R. Miles
MA, PhD, CPsychol, FBPsS

Those, if there are such, who still dispute the existence of dyslexia should read this book. John Osmond has described it as 'very much a layman's approach to the subject, by a concerned parent'. Layman's approach it may be, but to a professional such as myself it rings entirely true. Time and again I found myself saying, 'Yes, that is exactly the sort of thing that can happen.' It is distressing that there are still people in high places for whom the pattern of difficulties in dyslexia – as outlined in this book and elsewhere – is not obvious.

This means that families sometimes have to deal not just with the difficulties which arise from the dyslexia itself but with the frustration of unsatisfactory negotiations with officialdom. John Osmond's struggles to obtain proper help for Tomos are vividly documented in the first chapter of this book. But how many other Tomoses are there who have not been so lucky?

Dyslexia is of course a nuisance but if it is sympathetically handled it need not be a calamity. It is a calamity only if the difficulties are compounded by lack of understanding. In my experience this lack of understanding takes two main forms. In the first place, if dyslexic children are not told the nature of their difficulties they readily come to believe that they are 'thick' or 'stupid'; and it is clearly very frustrating to find that other children can easily cope with tasks which they themselves find difficult. The resultant uncertainty and loss of confidence is sometimes increased by insensitive remarks from teachers. Such teachers would never for an instant mock at or adversely criticize a physically disabled or deaf child, but if they have not been alerted to the needs of dyslexic children – and to the likelihood of an uneven performance – it is all too easy for them to assume that such children are lazy or 'playing up'. Secondly, there can be distressing consequences for parents. In particular – and this has happened many, many times in my experience – they are given the impression that they are being over-fussy or over-protective. In the case of a dyslexic child the advice 'Don't worry; she (he) is a late developer – it will come' is disastrous. None of us likes to be thought of as over-fussy or over-protective; and the consequence can be – as it was in Tomos Osmond's case – that valuable time is wasted before suitable help is obtained. When I myself talk to parents I encourage them to use common sense and to trust their own judgement.

If it is suspected that a child aged five or six – or even younger – is dyslexic then the organizing of suitable help cannot possibly do harm; in particular there is every reason to encourage children to learn the sounds made by individual letters of the alphabet. Then, if they turn out to have no major reading or spelling problems so much the better. It is the 'false negative' that is disastrous – the *denial* that a dyslexic child is dyslexic. All too often parents of ten- and eleven-year-olds have said to me, 'I knew since he was about six that there was something puzzling about him, but I was told not to fuss and that he would grow out of it.' In such cases sympathetic understanding could have saved years of frustration and discouragement, while 'catching up' on reading and spelling would have been correspondingly easier.

I should like to end this Foreword with three comments on the political scene.

In the first place, it is sometimes argued that 'lack of resources' – in other words, shortage of money – prevents proper help being given. It should be pointed out, however, that if an undiagnosed dyslexic sits at the back of the class learning nothing, this is in itself a terrible waste of resources – the more so since it is now realized that dyslexics sometimes have exceptional talents, for instance in art or engineering. It has recently been suggested that these talents may come even more to the fore now that computers can do so many of the clerical 'chores' that used to be done by scribes (see Thomas West's book, *In the Mind's Eye: Gifted People with Learning Difficulties, Computer Images, and the Ironies of Creativity*, published in 1991 by Prometheus Books, New York). Moreover the wastage is not just in the educational field: there may be demands on the health service and, alas!, on the prison service which are the direct consequence of our collective failure to give dyslexics the help and understanding that they need. It is absurd that education officers should be put in a position where they have to say, 'Because we do not have £x now it will be necessary to spend £50x of public money later,' and it is even more absurd that they should have to say, 'The prison service budget is nothing to do with *us*.' The issue of virement between budgets is one which I believe politicians and civil servants could tackle if the will were there.

Secondly, national testing of seven-year-olds in literacy skills need not necessarily be a bad thing provided it is sensitively handled. If it is undertaken solely with the aim of finding out who needs extra help and if an ethos is built up such that 'needing extra help' in any area is not regarded as a stigma, it could be welcomed. Sadly, however, there are all kinds of pressures which may lead to something different. If the assumption on the part of teachers and pupils is that tests are something which you 'pass' or 'fail', then for the dyslexic there will be an overwhelming fear of failure. If league tables are published comparing different schools there may be pressures not to accept dyslexics as they may lower one's school's rating; and if they are accepted there may still be teachers who suppose that they themselves are to blame for the dyslexic's literacy problems. If blame is to be attached at all (and often the mishandling of dyslexics arises from ignorance rather than malice), it should be directed at those who show insensitivity and an unwillingness to listen.

Finally, a further word on league tables. Some friendly rivalry between institutions is perhaps harmless, but to assume that competitiveness should play a major part in motivating teachers to give of their best is to promote a demeaning view of human nature. In addition it seems to me that appalling harm can be done to the morale of teachers in those schools which undeservedly receive a 'low' rating. The criteria for grading may well be in dispute, and the injustice inflicted on dedicated workers has not, in my view, been taken seriously enough. It is, of course, agreed that league tables would be more meaningful if a 'value added' factor were included, so that organizations could be judged not by some absolute standard but by what they did within the constraints imposed on them. For this reason it seems important – if there have to be league tables – that there should be bonus points for those schools which accept dyslexics and achieve success with them. Better still, however, it is to be hoped that governing bodies of schools will give a higher priority to helping children in need than to worrying about the position of their school in league tables.

All these issues, and more, are raised by John Osmond's excellent book, and I would beg all those who make educational decisions to take his arguments seriously.

T. R. MILES
Bangor, 1993

Acknowledgements

My first and main debt in writing this book has been to all those dyslexic people named in these pages who have given so freely of their time and experiences. It is a hopeful sign that they have been so willing to discuss openly what in the past has often been clouded by shame, secrecy and ignorance.

I am grateful, too, to the many professionals who have offered their advice, in particular to Professor Tim Miles who has contributed the Foreword to this book, Lee Pascal, Louise Green, Elizabeth Richards, Dr Uta Frith, Cynthia Klein, Carolyn Moran, Janice Edwards, Maryrose Crossman, Janet Tod and Jill Hutchings. Jean Augur, Ann Brereton and Charlie Griffiths at the British Dyslexia Association, and Jennifer John of my own South Wales Dyslexia Association, were a constant support.

In passing, the preponderance of women in the above list reflects a fundamental reality concerning dyslexia, immediately obvious to anyone who attends meetings about it around the country. This is that it is women who are most concerned and involved, as mothers, teachers and in support generally. And this is despite the fact that it is men more than women who are affected by dyslexia, by a factor of four to one.

The idea for this book grew out of research I undertook for a television documentary on dyslexia, made by Poseidon Films and first transmitted on Channel 4 and S4C in March 1993. The producer, Frixos Constantine, was an inspiration and the director, Paul Morrison, discovered many new avenues. I am grateful to

Gwynn Pritchard who, as the commissioning editor at Channel 4, first put me in touch with the project.

Naomi Roth at Cassell was at all times positive and forbearing in equal proportions. As ever my wife Alphie provided much detailed editorial help and encouragement.

My greatest debt in this project, however, is to my son Tomos Rhys who has taught me most of what I know about dyslexia. As he said a long time ago, the best way to spell 'because' is to say to yourself, 'Big elephants can always undress small elephants.' Our thanks go to his teacher and friend, Liz Twose, responsible for such essential strategies and much else besides.

Chapter 1

Living with Dyslexia

It has been dubbed the 'middle-class disease' and that is certainly the way we were made to feel about it when we first wondered whether our six-year-old son, Tomos, might be dyslexic. The symptoms were common enough. He was extremely slow at reading, his handwriting looked like hieroglyphics, and he was generally behind what you would expect for his age. He was in the remedial group in the class, but in other ways appeared bright, and of at least average intelligence.

Things were complicated because he was attending a Welsh-medium school, one of a growing number in Wales in which children are taught through the medium of the Welsh as well as the English language. So Tomos was having to cope with two languages. Could that be it? We saw his teacher, his headmaster, then an educational psychologist. Tests were done. His hearing was all right, despite the fact that he had suffered from glue ear when he was a toddler and had had his adenoids removed. He was of above average intelligence. Yes, certainly he was behind his age in attainment, but so were lots of children. It was too early to judge.

Dyslexic? 'We prefer not to use the term,' said the educationalists. 'We refer to specific learning difficulty. Anyway it's far too early to tell. He's a good-natured child, very willing and co-operative. We're sure he'll come on. Give him time.' That's exactly what we did: two years in fact. Looking back they were wasted years. For after that time had elapsed things were pretty much the same. By now Tomos was eight, had moved to another

Welsh-medium school, and had hardly opened a book, let alone read one. By his age his older sister had been an avid reader.

Instead Tomos watched endless television, and was still receiving 'remedial' help. By now he was beginning to learn English and when we saw his writing in his school books we really began to worry. His spelling was all over the place, with the letters jumbled up. Rather than needing to correct his spelling you felt you had to crack a code.

So we went back to the school and this time the reception was different. At least one of the teachers, the remedial teacher, was worried. She agreed that Tomos should be making more progress but was at a loss to explain why he was not. At our insistence we went once more to the educational psychologist for yet more tests: 'Yes, Tomos is of above average intelligence,' we were told. 'Yes, he should be given special help with reading.'

But dyslexia? 'Well, you know, that's a very controversial area . . . .' It turned out that this particular educational psychologist was sceptical about the notion, co-author of a book challenging the idea that it is a discrete condition separate from the more general area of reading backwardness.

So we took Tomos to the Dyslexia Unit at the University College of North Wales, Bangor, to see an acknowledged expert who worked there, Professor Tim Miles. After more tests he pronounced that he was in no doubt that Tomos was dyslexic. His report noted that Tomos showed the 'classic signs' of dyslexia which occur where there is relatively high ability yet strikingly weak spelling.

Professor Miles's report continued:

> Dyslexia implies a constitutionally caused anomaly of development (in no way Tomos's fault) which makes the acquisition of language skills – including spelling in particular – more difficult. It is therefore essential that he receives special help, particularly with reading, spelling, and the basics of numbers, if he is to make proper use of his other abilities.
>
> It is also essential that the teacher should understand the precise nature of the dyslexic's difficulties and be willing to use the structured, multisensory approach which is known to be effective in the great majority of cases. For most economical use of the specialist teacher's time I recommend the use of phonic check lists (so that reading and spelling can be improved concurrently), for instance

from *Alpha to Omega* (Honsby and Shear) and/or *Help for Dyslexic Children* (Miles and Miles).

After discussion with Professor Miles we moved Tomos to an English-medium school where he would only have to cope with learning to spell in one language. He began to receive one-to-one help in school from a remedial teacher but one not trained in dyslexic techniques. So we paid for Tomos to have private tuition for an hour a week from a specially trained dyslexia teacher who provided us with a programme of work to do daily at home. This we did for half an hour each morning before Tomos went to school.

Tomos hated all the extra work, which he found tiring. But he persevered and made rapid progress. In a little more than a year he moved from being a year behind his chronological age in reading and three years behind in spelling, to being slightly ahead in reading, and only a year behind in spelling.

This is an example of a piece of writing soon after Tomos began his programme of special help and extra work (the handwriting was neat since Tomos took a painfully long time over it):

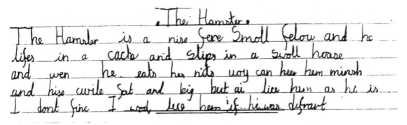

The Hamster

The Hamster is a nise fere Small felow and he lifes in a cache and slips in a swoll hoase and wen he eats hes nits uoy can heer hem minsh and hise cwile Sat and big but ai lice him as hi is I dont finc I wod lic hem if hi was difrart

This is an example of a piece of writing a year later:

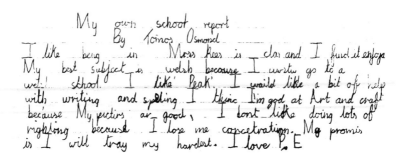

My own schoot report
By Tomos Osmond

I like beng in Mrss Rees is clas and I find it enjoyale. My best subject is welsh because I uwstw go to a welsh school. I like PeaK. I woild like a bit of help with writing and speling. I thinc I'm god at Art and craft because My pictirs ar good. I dont like doing lots of righting because I lose me concetration. My promis is I will tray my hardest. I love P.E

This progress nearly turned out to be our undoing. When Tomos began receiving special help in school the local education authority suggested we apply for a Statement to be made by the authority under the 1981 Education Act identifying his special educational needs. The advantage would be that henceforward, throughout his school career, Tomos would be regularly monitored and that extra help would be provided when necessary. It would also be easier for him to be allowed extra time to sit his examinations in secondary school.

So we applied for the Statement and Tomos was subjected to yet more tests, from teachers, doctors and educational psychologists. Meanwhile, when we had moved him to his new English-medium school we had placed him in a class a year younger than age group. In fact the difference was not very great since Tomos's birthday falls near the end of the school year, in June. Even so, the result was that he had more time to adjust and to catch up.

Assessing him for a Statement and waiting for the decision took more than a year. When the decision came it was that the LEA had decided against because, it said, Tomos was now at a reading age approximately that of his chronological age. To us this betrayed a view that somehow Tomos's problems had been 'solved', that he would need no further help and support. So we appealed against the LEA's decision, to the Welsh Office where the Secretary of State is responsible for education within Wales.

This entailed yet more tests and another wait of a year. In the event the Welsh Office agreed with us and ordered the local education authority to reconsider its decision. This it did, testing Tomos yet again, and then presented us with a bombshell. Because he had made such progress, the authority said, we should now move him up a form so that he would be in his 'correct' chronological age group.

We were very worried by this prospect. It was being suggested, we felt, not in Tomos's best interests but to provide the local education authority with extra ammunition to confront the Welsh Office. As far as Tomos was concerned a move could be disastrous. He had only just settled down in his new class and made friends. We knew that although he was making progress, it was fragile. He would always find reading, writing and spelling a painful chore and in any event they were still below the level we felt he was capable of achieving. The tests the experts employed seemed artificial and did not to us, who live with Tomos day to day, reflect his real social and emotional needs.

Our main concern was the impact a move would have on Tomos emotionally. It would mean him missing the final class in primary school and, cutting away from his new-found friends and peer group, moving straight into secondary school. That change is difficult enough for all children. But to inflict it on a dyslexic child a year sooner than expected, and without his friends, seemed to us a bizarre suggestion. We felt it was prompted by an education authority anxious to defend its position against central government and concerned too that making a Statement for a moderately dyslexic child like Tomos would establish a precedent with unforeseen financial implications.

So we fought the decision. We took Tomos to an independent educational psychologist and subjected him to further tests. These were more comprehensive than those that had been carried out by the local education authority. This time it was found that Tomos's reading level was three months behind his chronological age, but actually eight months lower than what could reasonably be expected from his IQ scores. While his comprehension was six months better than could be expected, he was about eighteen months behind in spelling. On the proposed move into secondary school the educational psychologist concluded that this would place Tomos 'at an emotional and academic disadvantage'.

In our campaign to have Tomos Statemented we elicited the support of his private dyslexia teacher, Elizabeth Twose, who wrote:

> It seems that Tomos is in a catch-22 situation, due to the fact that his parents are:
>
> (a) articulate and intelligent enough to explore all avenues in their quest to obtain the help appropriate for their son;
> (b) able to afford to pay for private tuition for him.
>
> Because of this Tomos's spelling and reading ages have improved so significantly that the Education Authority claim they have no need 'to make special educational provision' for him. Had his parents not persisted and obtained specialist help for Tomos it is unlikely that his reading and spelling age would have improved so significantly. He would then have been eligible for statementing under the criteria apparently being adopted by the Education Authority.

Professor Miles wrote, 'Unless he is Statemented I am puzzled to see how his special needs can be met.'

In the event the education authority still refused to make a Statement. However, it relented over forcing Tomos to move out of his class and so, prematurely from his point of view, enter secondary school a year earlier than expected.

Though Tomos is dyslexic he is not severely dyslexic. He has managed to cope, with a great deal of support, within the school system. Yet if he had not been identified (against the odds as it happened) as dyslexic and received appropriate help he would have been stranded at school. He would have been labelled a backward child, and undoubtedly become a failure in terms of conventional measurements such as passing examinations. So Tomos has been lucky. Many other children in his position are not.

WHAT IS DYSLEXIA?

This book is mainly about the experiences of dyslexic people: children, adults and also families because there are strong indications that dyslexic characteristics are genetically linked, and so run in families. It is aimed especially at parents who suspect their children may be suffering from dyslexia and at teachers who want to find out more. The reason for the emphasis is that there is great difficulty in appreciating what dyslexia feels like if you do not suffer from it yourself.

Unlike many obviously physical handicaps you cannot see dyslexia. Moreover dyslexia is not a straightforward condition which you either have or do not have in a straightforward, objective sense. Every dyslexic person, being by definition an individual, experiences dyslexia in his or her own particular way. It is best to think of dyslexia as experienced along a spectrum from mild to severe. The one thing all dyslexics tend to have in common is much higher than average levels of anxiety.

The word dyslexia comes from the Greek language and its literal translation is *dys* – difficulty, *lexis* – words: hence, difficulty with words, difficulty with reading, spelling, written prose and sometimes arithmetic. It is estimated that some 60 per cent of dyslexics have difficulty with numeracy.

Dyslexia occurs in spite of normal teaching and is independent of socio-cultural background or intelligence. In fact, far from being a 'middle-class disease' dyslexia occurs in people across the same class and intelligence range as the rest of the population.

A dyslexic person may also have difficulties with orientation (for example, distinguishing between left and right), time, short-term memory (auditory or visual), sequencing, auditory or visual perception and motor skills. Many specialists speak of a 'pattern of difficulties'.

At least one person in twenty-five is dyslexic to some extent. Perhaps 2 per cent of the population can be counted as suffering from severe dyslexia. These statistics mean that in most classrooms there will be at least one dyslexic child, if not two.

Dyslexia is more easily detected in those with average or above average intelligence because of the obvious difference between their literacy skills and intelligence and abilities in other spheres. This leads directly to one of the main hazards of dealing with dyslexia in schools. Many dyslexics do learn to read quite competently in spite of their handicap, overcoming their difficulties by themselves. As a result they can go unnoticed and fail to reach their full potential. For many people a dyslexic who can read adequately is seen as a contradiction in terms.

The experience of a dyslexic person is analogous to the aerial on a television being not quite focused on the transmitter. The television itself is in perfect working order, but the sounds and images it receives get blurred. So a dyslexic might write or read *was* for saw, or *dos* or *dose* for does.

Most dyslexic children have difficulties with phonological processing, that is, managing and memorizing sequences of the speech sounds whose relationship to print forms the basis of learning to read. This includes skills in relation to rhymes (*hot, pot*), segmentation (*hope-less*), blending (*s-i-t* becomes *sit*) and phonemes (*bright* without *r* makes *bite*). This phonological processing is precisely the aspect of literacy that turns out to be the most genetically determined.

Dyslexics do not hear sounds or see images in the normal way. For dyslexics, to be told to look at a word and learn it is often simply impossible. When they first look at a word it is typically seen as a jumble of letters, an incoherent mixture of shapes that somehow have to be perceived as a sensible pattern. At the start a dyslexic just doesn't know how to begin to *learn* it.

To get an idea, describe to yourself, without looking, what exactly is on the face of your watch. Remember that this is an object you must have looked at a thousand times. Does it have Roman numerals, letters, a date, a minute hand . . . ? Or try drawing a symbol you will have seen many times, say the British Rail logo or the disability sign.

What this should reveal is that we don't learn merely by looking. There is also what is termed a kinaesthetic dimension to learning: recognition by shape and touch. This is important for all of us but especially so for dyslexic people. To get a sense of this simply close your eyes and write your name on a piece of paper, without looking. Then, without looking again, write the word *constabulary*.

There is little doubt that you will not have had to sound out your own name as you wrote it. Your hand will have flowed automatically, working with the kinaesthetic memory. The same would apply to changing gears in a car, or tying your shoelaces. These are actions which require little conscious thought.

So it is with spelling. Some words are so familiar that we can visualize them without thinking, operating by auditory, kinaesthetic memory. This applies for example to a word like *house*. But a word like *constabulary* creates difficulties. We are not so familiar with it and so have to find a different way of 'receiving' it, perhaps by spelling it out verbally to ourselves.

People who are not dyslexic tend to assume that the visual sense will work by itself. And for most of the time it does. For dyslexics, however, the visual sense is often not the most reliable. They have to find other methods. So, for instance, writing down notes is not a pedagogically sound method for learning as far as dyslexics are concerned. For them, writing things down once doesn't satisfy the kinaesthetic requirement.

If you wanted to teach someone from scratch how to tie their shoelaces you wouldn't rely on just visual or auditory methods by themselves. The same applies doubly and to a far greater range of things to dyslexics. Continually they have to discover extra dimensions than simply the visual to receive and store information, let alone recall it. So, for example, joined-up writing is helpful for dyslexics. It can provide flow and maturity to words and make their spelling 'feel' right.

Lee Pascal, an inspirational London-based teacher of dyslexics, refers to his own disability – colour blindness – when explaining what dyslexia is like. 'My colour blindness is divorced from intellectual problems,' he says.

> It is a perceptual difficulty. I cannot tell the difference between red, brown and green. No matter how hard I concentrate I cannot discriminate between these colours. So, for example, as far as I'm concerned I have fourteen pairs of black socks.
>
> It is the same with dyslexics. If they get their *b*s and *d*s confused it is no use shouting at them, *Concentrate!*
>
> In my case, when I was a child I had all my pencils marked with the appropriate colour named on them. My teacher found a solution. She didn't shout *Concentrate!* or *Focus harder!*

'SORRY, IT'S A DYSLEXIC DAY'

The consequences of simply shouting at dyslexic people, of failing to understand their problems and what it feels like to have them, are simply to compound their frustration. Even worse, it is to increase their very large potential for low self-esteem and even humiliation. The following is how one forty-year-old dyslexic woman expressed it:

> Do you suffer daily embarrassment or humiliation? I do! My humiliation is a difficult thing to write about because every word I use could compound that humiliation: My Huemillyashon!

The feeling can rear its ugly head when you least expect it and it usually does. One could be talking to friends, shopping or at a meeting. It can happen at absolutely any time or in any place. To trigger it off only requires a situation that calls for me to write. The more unexpected the situation, the more public the time, the greater will be the humiliation.

What do you say when a seven-year-old asks you to spell a word for him, because his teacher is busy? What do you say when you have to write a cheque but cannot spell the name? What do you say when a group of friends say, 'Let's play a quiz game'? What do you say when at a meeting you are asked to take names? What do you say when the headmaster of your children's school says, 'Leave a note on my desk', and you cannot even remember how to spell his name?

You could say, 'I have forgotten my glasses', or 'I haven't got a pen', or you could say, 'I can't spell!' If only that simple explanation would suffice. Most people will not accept that an adult of average intellect really cannot use the written English language accurately. They think you mean you cannot spell complex words; they do not realize that a five-letter word could hold five pitfalls for you.

I have lived with this humiliation, frustration and embarrassment for forty years and though it does get easier to deal with, it is always there just waiting to strike.

I was six or seven when I first began to have special lessons. How I hated those dreaded weekly appointments. Each week a few of us would leave our own classroom for a lesson in the headmaster's office. I can remember to this day the smell of stale smoke and see the semi-circle of small chairs around his large, brown desk. It was not just the lessons I detested but the disappointment of what I had missed back in the classroom. All through my school life I was helped, always without success. At school I could not escape from writing, therefore I could not escape from humiliation.

I chose an occupation that I thought would not require me to write but as my career progressed I was put under increasing pressure to write. A 'kind' personnel officer once said to me, 'Don't worry, I have a dictionary in my desk if you need it.' I could have told her, 'I never go anywhere without one in my bag. It's one in my head I need.'

I have given much time in recent years to spelling classes without any marked success. The lessons did not teach me to spell but I did learn to be honest in most situations and say, 'Help, I can't spell!' There are no lessons to help cope with the humiliation that those words conjure up.

If only there was a magic tablet I could have taken to make my brain retain all the hundreds of words I have learnt thousands of times. Most people learn a word and they have got it for life but not me and many like me. We learn the same word over and over again, but when that word is needed our minds go blank or the letters come out in the wrong order.

I liken my brain to a sponge. I dip it in the water of knowledge, take it out, I can spell! Leave it for a day or two and slowly, drip by drip, that knowledge seeps away and I am back searching for all those lost words.

There is more to not being able to spell than the embarrassment and humiliation. There is the frustration of never being able to write a quick note, be it a message to an employer or a letter excusing a child from school. For even these basic forms of communication require time: time to write the note in rough, time to find the dictionary, time to correct, time to write an acceptable copy.

Often you cannot find a word in the dictionary if you cannot spell it, so you have to rethink the whole sentence . . . more wasted time and frustration.

If I had 10p for every time I asked God to deliver me from a situation or inspire me with the letters I need, hopefully in the right order, I would be a rich woman. No one can really comprehend another person's humiliation. No one can really know how I feel when I cannot carry out what is considered by most as a simple adult task, to write a word using the correct letters in the right order.

Louise Green is another dyslexic in her forties whose family of three dyslexic children is profiled in Chapter 4. She discovered she was dyslexic when she was thirty-three, after her oldest child had been diagnosed when he was eight years old. She has an IQ of 158, well above the 100 average. Here she describes her own upbringing, schooling and early career:

I can remember, from a very young age, not being able to follow instructions clearly and then getting into trouble. For example, one Christmas when I was about three I asked if I could do some drawing and on being told that I could use the old telephone directory, somehow managed to misunderstand which one that was, thereby ruining the brand new one.

Another time I remember spending an agonizingly long time sewing a dress for my doll, only to have the whole lot fall apart because I had somehow missed the bit about tying a knot.

I got into trouble frequently for not following instructions because it was obvious that I was an intelligent child and my parents just assumed I was naughty or attention seeking, especially as I was in the middle of five – later six – children. I can clearly remember being unhappy because I was 'naughty' but not realizing that true naughtiness is when a child deliberately does something wrong.

I had assumed that naughtiness was just something I was born with, like having fair hair, something beyond my control. In spite of having a happy home life, with fair-minded and loving parents, even today I can remember the terrible feelings of sickening dread, isolation and being totally misunderstood that periodically would sweep over me when yet again I had done something 'wrong', unintentionally.

As I got older and was given more responsibilities, these lapses, these 'misunderstandings' got worse. On one occasion all my brothers and sisters waited for over two hours for me at the bus-stop nearest our home because I was waiting for them to arrive at my end of the bus route so we could travel home together. My mother never did understand that I honestly thought that was what she had meant and that I wasn't being stupid, naughty or tiresome.

Something I dreaded that cropped up time and again was when a member of my family expected me to remember a person or event by name. When I couldn't, they would get very cross/annoyed/irritated with me and insist that I did or must remember. To avoid further grilling, and so as not to appear stupid, I would pretend that suddenly I understood what they were talking about and, of course, I remembered.

One of the worst occasions was when my youngest brother was born and given a name I had not heard before. It seemed to take weeks to learn an apparently unrelated collection of syllables that everyone else knew. It left me feeling very insecure, for if everyone else could do things that I couldn't (or was it really *wouldn't*?) then it *must* be my fault.

From then on, until I discovered my dyslexia in later life, I used to apologize for everything around me, even if someone stepped on *my* toe. Even today I feel sick inside when I'm told that someone wants to talk to me or see me.

Problems seemed to begin in my second year in school. I was told off for things I didn't understand and therefore didn't know I was doing wrong. I was punished by having to miss art and other 'fun' lessons to do the work again. I know the other children thought I was stupid and they teased me.

One afternoon I even ran away, although that too appeared to be all my fault. I thought (and still believe) that the teacher told me that if I was late again, she would send me home. The next day I was late and when the teacher pointed to the classroom door I thought she was telling me to go home. So I went, crying all the way. The teacher later explained that she had wanted me to get the register from another classroom.

The next school year was even worse. Luckily I could remember my tables and was good at sums, but reading and spelling were a nightmare. Even if I had learned the wretched spellings by rote, by the next day they had totally vanished from my brain. I survived by cheating, copying from a friend or writing the answers lightly and going over them afterwards. This failed the day the teacher gave us the wrong list and I could not erase the original answers.

I don't remember being taught phonic sounds at all, but I do remember being told all about the magic 'e' and not understanding a word of it. I think I put an 'e' at the end of every word for the next few weeks.

Reading wasn't much better. I learned to 'read' by memorizing whole chunks of the books I was given and as long as I could see the pictures I would be all right. The frustrating thing was that while I could understand most of the book I could not verbalize many of the actual words. The strategy fell apart the day the teacher turned two pages by mistake and I did not notice. She did.

At eight I changed schools and had a horrendous time. At the old school we called the teacher 'Miss'. At the new school we were expected to call the teacher by name. Although I knew we should do this, even so I kept calling the teacher 'Miss' because I couldn't remember her real name. It was a collection of syllables I had not heard before and which did not sound like any other word I knew at the time.

By now it was obvious that though I was in the top set for Maths I was hopeless at spelling, reading and writing. My handwriting was awful, work was careless and apparently I was a lazy little girl who could do better if only she would try harder. Reports like this haunted me throughout my school career and deep down I still believe that I am a lazy, careless person in spite of all the evidence to the contrary.

I still had problems reading aloud because I couldn't remember how words were pronounced even if I knew what they meant. The books I read for pleasure were all meant for children younger than myself. My reading only improved when I discovered the Andrew Lang series of fairy-tales at eleven. Because I adored the stories I persevered and went from these on to the Hornblower novels by C. S. Forrester. I caught up with children's fiction when I was at college.

I failed my eleven-plus exam and felt devastated. I had gone for extra tests because I was borderline but I misread the essay title and wrote about a day on the beach in high summer instead of about a day in the *winter* holidays. I can still remember the panic I felt when I realized what I'd done and tried to rewrite it.

French was the only secondary school subject I loathed. Although I was all right at the written work, I could not read French aloud without translating it into English in my head, turning that back into French and saying the words from memory, not from what was printed on the page. Generally I had a problem remembering French words unless I could link them to a 'sound-alike' word I already knew.

Spelling was still my major problem and the work I had to put in was astronomical. Our final form position depended on the total of all our exam results so every term I had to relearn all the spellings we'd been given so far. By the summer term I was learning from scratch over three hundred spellings as I never remembered them from before. I never once got full marks.

I baffled my secondary school teachers. They could see I was one of the most able pupils in the school and yet I still made 'careless' mistakes. Although no adult had ever accused me of stupidity, I thought that I wasn't very clever and was just lucky to get good marks, often wondering whether the staff were upgrading my work to be kind to me.

No one, least of all myself, realized that I had a specific learning difficulty. Teachers tried a variety of ways to counter my 'careless-ness', including ridicule (which still makes me cringe today), such as being laughed at by the whole class at sixteen because I'd written *scarf* as *scraf* and couldn't see the mistake.

With age and experience I worked out or invented strategies to overcome many of my difficulties, including revision skills. I used to read through my notes, make brief headings with numbered sub-points and learn these. I tested myself by reciting or trying to rewrite these key points.

This strategy backfired on me quite badly when I was fifteen. As I kept coming top in most subjects, the rest of the class assumed I was cheating and when they found my revision notes they thought they had proof. But the only times I had cheated were to help my friends with their answers.

I got eight good O levels, in spite of misreading the instructions on one English paper and answering far too many questions. I then moved schools to take three A levels. Here the problems were different. My spelling was still erratic, although not so noticeable, and reading aloud was a thing of the past. However, I lacked many of the necessary study skills for successfully tackling A level course work and took a very long time working out exactly what they were.

Eventually I got three A levels and went to university. I opted to do Biblical Studies because I didn't think I'd get a place reading History. However, as part of the course I had to learn Greek and Hebrew. I couldn't cope with the Greek and left at the end of the first term to go into teaching, because I was afraid I wouldn't be able to complete the university course. I managed my way through teacher training college and got my teaching certificate.

Teaching was often a fraught experience, especially at first. Remembering the names of the children was difficult, and virtually impossible when they were ones I had never heard before. Correcting work was difficult, too, since I was never sure of the spellings myself. Blackboard work was a minefield and I had to be careful over what I actually wrote. Once I wrote *public* without the *l* in front of a mixed twelve-year-old class. I knew I'd made a mistake because of the smothered giggles but I couldn't see it. Another teacher had to point it out.

Reading aloud became a problem again. As class teacher I had to read an ongoing story at least once a week. I couldn't read accurately, frequently transposing words and occasionally reaching a word that I couldn't remember how to pronounce. When these lapses occurred I would either substitute a word with one having a similar meaning or else stop dead and stare around the classroom as if someone had been misbehaving, giving myself 'thinking' time.

Once a pupil was following me in a copy of the book and wanted to know why I didn't read exactly what was printed. I hurriedly assured him that I kept losing my place because I had to keep checking on class behaviour. Luckily that seemed to satisfy him, but it left me feeling inadequate that an eleven-year-old could read better than I could.

Jennie Peel, who lives in West Sussex, brought up two sons, the youngest one a dyslexic, but only discovered that she herself was dyslexic when he was twelve and she forty-two. She recalls how it happened:

I was sitting at a meeting organized by our local dyslexia association, listening to Professor Tim Miles talking about *Research and the Older Dyslexic* and was suddenly hit by one of his comments. It was something like, 'You and I would be able to do so and so, but a dyslexic would find it difficult.'

From that moment things began to fall into place, and I began to understand why so many things had been the way they had. Since then I've read practically every book on the reading list about dyslexia, learnt so much, and realized . . . Yes, me too!

I was just so lucky. My first teacher, when I was four and a half, insisted that all her pupils would read before they went on to the next year. As I remember we did not do anything else until we had learnt and I was the last. However, she had the maxim 'if one way doesn't work we'll try another'. I remember so clearly her writing 'Sam the Pig' and turning it into a picture. The blasted grapes Sam ate are forever embellished on my brain!

There were lots of pictures, games, all the sorts of teaching now recommended by experts. I was reading by the time I was six.

At seven I went to the Elmhurst Ballet School in Camberley. Many of my companions there are now in the theatre, dancing schools, or film and television studios around the world, and I suspect that very many of us were dyslexic. Did the word exist then?

It was a professional training school for classical ballet and drama, but of course we had to do the usual boring old things like Maths and Geography. Writing was very important and we were given beautifully written 'pieces'. When we could reproduce one to a high standard we would go on to the next. Mine was about some wretched King of Dunfermline and the Northern Lights. I never did get on to the next piece. In the end they just let me stop.

I was desperately keen to learn the piano when I was young. I always told everyone that I wanted to give up because we had to practise before breakfast in the dance studio and sometimes it was freezing. In reality it was because I found I couldn't read the music. I really did try hard, but apart from middle C it was useless. Later, when I was a student and we had to do *soubrette* song and dance I made intelligent comments about the rising crescendo (any fool could see the notes went up) and my friends taught me by ear, so no one ever knew.

I can remember sobbing through some lessons and being so frustrated because nothing seemed to 'go in'. I learnt punctuation by pretending I was acting: little breath equals a comma, big breath equals a full stop, and to hell with the semicolon!

The most important things as far as my peers were concerned were dance, art and drama. So I was far more fortunate than most dyslexics since I had something I could do well in. I firmly believed I was stupid, scatty and incapable of anything academic. Luckily this was acceptable in an 'arty' atmosphere. I can so well imagine how I would have felt if I was dependent on ordinary school subjects.

As it was I had very little self-confidence, poor self-esteem and I clowned around, sending myself up, before anyone else did. I can now see that I did have abilities and it was a lack of confidence in those abilities that held me back after I left school. I always had, and still have to a smaller degree, the feeling that I have to try to make up for my inadequacies.

I have always been clumsy, and even though a trained dancer, can fall over the only chair in an empty room. When I was a child we practically had a season ticket at the local hospital casualty unit as I was so accident prone. I have to allow 'getting lost' time when I go anywhere, even for the dozenth time. I have had some near misses on roundabouts for not giving way to the right which I could have sworn was the left.

I have had countless surprises when shopping. I know I bought chicken and sweetcorn soup, but it magicked itself into creamy Spanish onion by the time I got home. Perhaps the worst time was when I bought what I thought was some healthy wheatgerm for the family, only to find it was a special product for broody bitches.

Whenever I take a telephone number to ring someone back, I have learnt to tell them to ring me if they haven't heard by the appointed time. I have often spent hours ringing every combination of a six-figure number, as I seem to have written it down wrong.

I teach tap-dancing for evening classes, and nowadays don't even try to bluff when I have got in a complete muddle and can't remember what steps I've just set them. I just say, 'Sorry, it's a dyslexic day, let's try again.'

When I went to evening class to learn picture framing I felt all the old horrors returning. Everything was fine, until we came to using the ruler properly for the accuracy needed. I felt panic rising, my eyes started pricking, and those awful tears started forming. I didn't know what to do, and I was more than forty years old!

When the teacher, who was extremely kind and patient, came round I tried to bluff, couldn't, took a deep breath and said, 'I can't do it. I don't know how to use a ruler properly.' People didn't stare at me. Nobody shrieked with laughter. No one even noticed. The teacher explained, the panic subsided, and it was another step forward.

I first became consciously involved with dyslexia when my youngest son, Ben, had an unfortunately typical experience: us suggesting that all was not well, the school saying we were expecting too much, behavioural problems, and his being branded unteachable at eight years old. Eventually we had him assessed at the Dyslexia Institute. Hooray! Problem identified, now it can be solved. Or so we thought.

But the school disagreed: no help was available, there were endless difficulties and problems. When we finally got him organized at eleven years old, I decided that if I could just stop one child going through that appalling situation, mainly through people's ignorance of knowing what could be done, I would.

So I organized a meeting, to which nearly seventy people came. We started a local association, which is now affiliated to the British Dyslexia Association. I run a helpline, give talks to any group that will listen – the Rotary, playgroups and luncheon clubs – and give local radio interviews whenever I can think of a new angle.

I do voluntary learning support at our local comprehensive school. After going on at them about the need to help children with difficulties I thought I'd better put my money where my mouth was! It is sometimes a bit scary, though. Often I'm afraid of not following what the teacher is talking about since I certainly can't absorb a lot of the material first time round.

Supporting my son through his GCSEs was enormously time-consuming. He vowed he would leave school at the first possible opportunity, but having passsed six GCSEs, including English, he went on to do Sociology and Art at A level. Before helping Ben I hadn't realized that I read very fast to beat the 'jumping' of the print. It also made me realize that I was missing letters and sometimes whole words. Some days are worse than others, of course, as with most of what they call the symptoms.

Running the helpline brings it home to me that people are often misled by the emphasis on reading. I often get comments like, 'My son can't be dyslexic because he can read, but I'm so desperate . . .'.

I suppose if I had to pick one thing that is the biggest pain it would have to be the short-term memory, or the lack of it. This is one of the hardest things for others who haven't experienced it to understand.

I have had a varied, exciting and interesting time. It's getting even better, as I'm gradually becoming more self-confident inside. I could always manage to act the part, even when I was feeling like a tiny worm inside. But it's so much better not having to! I wish so much that I had known what the problem was years ago.

THE INHERITANCE FACTOR

Scattered through this book you will find comments from dyslexics like, 'Sometimes I feel like giving my brain a good wash', 'I read like my mouth doesn't belong to my brain', 'It's just like there's something in my brain that won't click open', 'My brain is back to front, really', or 'My hands don't do what my brain tells them to.' A thirty-two-year-old London man found to be dyslexic while serving a prison sentence for theft commented, 'The main benefit from improving my reading and writing skills would be writing my feelings down instead of keeping them locked in my head.'

The consistency of such remarks, from different people attempting to explain how they experience dyslexia, is strongly suggestive of what is becoming more and accepted as the explanation for the condition. This is that it is a genetically originated brain dysfunction. More often than not there is a family history of dyslexia; and boys seem to be affected more often than girls, by a ratio of three or four to one.

It remains the case, however, that the precise way dyslexia is inherited and the way its effects are transmitted through brain organization and signal transmission are shrouded in ignorance. Even in general terms the way the brain works is still relatively little understood. Yet some things are clear. The brain is split into two separate halves, a right and a left hemisphere. These communicate with each other by a long connecting set of nerve fibres. Although they look the same the two halves of the brain tend to perform different tasks. For most people the left side is the verbal, logical and controlling half, while the right is the non-verbal, practical, intuitive side. Thus, generally speaking it is the left hemisphere of the brain which processes language and communication. People also have a language area in the right side of their brain, but this is usually smaller and much less efficient in ordering and processing language-based skills.

Evidence is growing that dyslexic people tend to have the language areas of the two sides of their brains more or less equally split, with problems arising as a result in the processing of information. There is some suggestion too that dyslexics have to pass more messages from one hemisphere to another before linguistic symbols such as letters and numbers can be identified and named. It can follow therefore that dyslexics may experience a kind of traffic jam of messages between the two sides of the brain when language-based information is being absorbed, stored or transmitted.

This description is a highly simplified summary of a complex process which varies widely from individual to individual. None the less, its general thrust was confirmed in the early 1990s by research carried out at the National Institute of Child Health and Human Development in Washington, DC. This used a technique known as magnetic resonance imaging (MRI) to compare the brain structures of twenty-one dyslexics with those of twenty-nine normal readers.

The research showed that the rear portion of the brain's left hemisphere in normal readers was larger than the corresponding portion in the right hemisphere. In dyslexics, on the other hand, the rear portion of the left hemisphere was smaller than or the same size as the corresponding part of the right hemisphere. These findings have since been amplified by Professor Albert Galaburda of Boston, Massachusetts. He found through dissection distinct differences in the clusters of large cells in the areas of the brain which process visual and auditory information. Dyslexics had clusters roughly 30 per cent smaller than non-dyslexics of similar IQ. This suggests that for dyslexics processing detailed information quickly is a problem.

The brain differences between dyslexics and normal readers are not believed to be reflected in the overall performance and ability of their brains as such, for instance as measured by intelligence testing. All the evidence is that dyslexic people are distributed across the same range of intelligence as everybody else. And while dyslexic people plainly have problems in processing language together with other difficulties, this can be compensated for by enhanced attributes in other areas. For example, the brain structures of dyslexic people tend to provide them with a more holistic way of viewing the world, often reflected in artistic and other creative capabilities. That such diverse figures as Leonardo da Vinci, Auguste Rodin and Albert Einstein are all believed to have been dyslexic makes the point, one that is explored more fully in the final chapter.

As research work gradually yields more information some of the mists of ignorance surrounding dyslexia are lifting. In the process the weight of evidence is favouring those who have long argued that, though it is experienced in highly individual ways and along a spectrum of severity, dyslexia is a distinctive and recognizable condition. Further, it has its own particular causation, which requires it to be recognized, identified and dealt with as such, especially by educationalists.

In short, dyslexia is a reality whose denial has potential for enormous harm. Much of this potential for harm is reflected in the accounts and experiences of dyslexic people that are scattered through this book. Some of the consequences of failing to recognize and deal adequately with dyslexia will be discussed in the final chapter.

Although research into the physical causes of dyslexia is being pursued on a wide front, few believe that it will in any sense lead to a 'cure' for dyslexia. It should, however, result in better understanding, and more work on ways dyslexic people can be helped to cope with their difficulties. In any event, as Dr Harry Chasty, director of the Dyslexia Institute, has said, 'Rodin was dyslexic. Would we want to "cure" him? Part of his neurological organization was that he wasn't able to read, write or spell very well, but it produced those immensely wonderful sculptures.'

Chapter 2

Children

The worst problem any dyslexic has to face is not reading, writing or even spelling, but lack of understanding. This sometimes takes an extreme form when teachers, out of ignorance, can become even more frustrated than their pupils. Vanessa Howard, who was diagnosed as dyslexic when she was twelve, will never forget an incident that took place in the classroom of her Surrey school when she was eight years old. She had taken all morning to produce a painting but by the time she had finished she was certain it was the best she had ever done and took it to show her teacher at the front of the class.

'I was really proud of it,' she said. 'It was a field full of trees but the teacher took one look at it and ripped it up.' The painting was not what Vanessa had been asked to draw. 'I could never remember what she was saying,' Vanessa said. 'She labelled me slow and said I never paid attention. Sometimes she would tear up my writing because it was illegible. Every time I thought I'd done something good, she said it was rubbish. She just didn't know how to teach me.'

The impact of such incidents on children's self-esteem and self-confidence can be much more profoundly damaging than dyslexia itself. Even when dyslexic children have supportive and understanding teachers, there is always the chance that they will be bullied by other children or made to feel isolated in the classroom. For example, one ten-year-old child was chosen to read *Thomas the Tank Engine* out loud in class because this was the level he could manage. Henceforth, however, he was dubbed Thomas by the other children, who made 'choo choo' sounds whenever they saw him in the playground. Such treatment compounds the inherent frustration that afflicts all dyslexics and invariably at one time or another leads to temper tantrums, misbehaviour and even delinquency.

Parents know their children better than anyone else. If they think their child has a problem, then he or she probably has. Their difficulty, however, is that more often than not they have little idea where to turn for help. Moreover, there is as yet no consistency in the help that is available from one part of the country to another. If you are dyslexic life is a lottery, determined by the awareness, determination and financial circumstances of your parents, by the local education authority area into which you happen to be born, and by the attitude and awareness of the teachers you chance to meet.

Most of this chapter is made up of personalized accounts of the experiences of dyslexic children. They provide impressive evidence that once a proper diagnosis has been made and once effective support and teaching is under way at home and in the school, dyslexic children can cope with their difficulties. The alternative, which is failure to recognize the problem and failure to provide effective support, can lead to a downward spiral of low self-esteem. In turn this can often lead to effective withdrawal from the education process, anger and general resentment against the world, and inevitably the prospect of underachievement and a general sense of failure.

The following accounts provide an insight into the miserable life that can be endured by children whose dyslexia goes unrecognized. More than this, in the concluding chapter evidence will show that the frustrations dyslexic children experience can in some circumstances lead to delinquency and crime if they are not dealt with appropriately.

Even if a dyslexic child has the relative good fortune to be identified reasonably young and provided with effective help, this is not to say that his or her life will be easy. Christine Ostler, a teacher and a dyslexic herself, has written in her *Dyslexia: A Parents' Sur-* t there are no short cuts: 'I stress that children r dyslexia as an excuse,' she writes. 'To be told simply means that you must work much harder bour. They will often say that it is not fair, and

I explain that often life seems not to be fair but they have just got to get on with it.' It is interesting that Louise Green, another teacher and dyslexic, refers to the same point in Chapter 4, when discussing some of the trials of a family living with dyslexia. She adds, however, that this lesson of the essential unfairness of life can be an advantage when, as is invariably the case, dyslexics learn it early on.

Christine Ostler was prompted to write her book by the experiences of bringing up her dyslexic son, Jonathan. She says it was a tremendous advantage for her to have been dyslexic herself, because she had been through the processes of learning to laugh at some of the awful mistakes dyslexics inevitably make and had developed strategies to deal with them.

Even then it was not always straightforward, however.

> I remember trying to cheer Jonathan up on one occasion when he was about eight. He was very down about school and said he was no good at anything. I tried to reassure him that he was good at lots of things and that we knew he was trying his best. I added that it was not his fault that he found things difficult but that he had inherited his learning difficulties from me.
>
> That made him very angry and he blamed me for all his misfortunes. I call this the 'knife-in-the-stomach slowly twisting' syndrome. It lasted for about two years and it still upsets me to think how hard school was for him at that time. He knew in his heart that he wasn't stupid, but he wasn't old enough to be philosophical about the many frustrations he had to experience.

So, even with understanding and supportive parents, and even with effective help at school, life is far from easy for dyslexic children. It is much, much harder when these things do not apply.

PAUL DAVIS

Sylvia Davis never really recovered from the struggle to discover the nature of her son Paul's problem: so much so that, like many others who have been through the same experience, it changed her life. She became an activist, campaigning with local schools and councillors, first on behalf of her own son and later in support of other children. She became a founder member and secretary of the Hillingdon Dyslexia Association in London, one of many that have sprung up throughout Britain.

'When I first began to get anxious I was treated just as a fussy, middle-class mother by the primary school,' she said.

I was told that Paul was definitely not dyslexic. He was taught by a special needs teacher for a year but they still didn't believe anything was fundamentally wrong. They said he was a boy who didn't listen properly. They said dyslexia was such a rare condition that they had never had a child suffering from it in the school.

It was a response that at first sapped her confidence but in the end made her angry. Finally, when he was ten years old she took Paul to the the Dyslexia Institute in Staines where he was found to be dyslexic with an intellience quotient that put him among the top 10 per cent of the population. 'It was a great relief to all of us,' Sylvia Davis remembers. 'Paul said it felt like a great weight had been lifted from his shoulders. He said he had started to think he was going mad.'

Before he went to school Paul was quite advanced in many areas, such as drawing, making models and doing jigsaws. 'He was irritatingly good at undoing catches so that his pushchair straps had to be fastened and then knotted to keep him secure,' Sylvia recalled. 'In some ways he was an unusual little boy. I once found him in a pair of muddy wellingtons purposefully placing his feet around the inside of an empty bath. He had observed that his footprints made marks on the garden paving so he had carefully coated his boots with mud and then carried them upstairs to make patterns on the white enamel surface.'

Paul has always had an erratic memory and an extremely vague sense of time. 'One Christmas when he was about seven years old, I remember going through the usual Christmas Eve ritual of excitedly hanging up his stocking at the end of the bed,' said Sylvia. 'Next morning we were surprised when he didn't come rushing into our bedroom. On investigation we found him sitting on his bedroom floor quietly building Lego models. His stocking was untouched because he had completely forgotten it was Christmas Day.'

At nursery school his teacher commented on the detailed work he put into model-making and said he had an unusually good memory for his age. However, he was one of the last children to be given a reading book because he couldn't master the pre-reading exercises, and that was when Sylvia's unease began. She gave up her work as a librarian to be at home with Paul and spent a lot of time reading to him.

'Although he certainly loved books, he would always start yawning and rubbing his eyes when he had to read something himself,' she said.

It was clear that his real interest was in mechanical objects. For instance he would thoroughly enjoy investigating the workings of an old radio.

He liked to sleep with a collection of wires and batteries under his pillow and his pockets were similarly full of unusual items. Paul would sit on a crowded train and, to the amazement of fellow passengers, occupy himself with the pliers, lengths of chain and suchlike that he always carried with him.

He once insisted on packing his own bag when visiting his grandmother for a weekend and she told me later that he had forgotten his swimming trunks but had included a whole load of plumbing equipment.

Paul's burglar alarms plagued his family from when he was about eight years old. They encompassed a range of design. One memorable contraption featured a large balloon which was attached to a door by string and elastic. It would deflate when the door was opened, thereby expelling the air through a strategically placed whistle. Another was linked to a stereo system so that deafening music would blast the eardrums of an unfortunate intruder.

The family also had to put up with cable-cars across the living room and a mechanical milk-shake mixer in the kitchen. This last gadget was constructed from Lego-technic and on high-speed setting could propel the contents of a glass across a remarkably wide area. Other devices included a bird-feeding machine, a moth-trap and self-closing bedroom cupboards. Paul developed something of the character of a mad inventor, with a 'Privet – Keep Out!' sign on his bedroom door.

There was a very different picture at school, however. 'The happy, bubbly boy we saw at home was very different from the daydreaming child who struggled in the classroom,' said his mother.

Paul was almost ten years old when I found him crying over a spelling list. He explained that words seemed to move around when he tried to read, that he couldn't copy anything because he was unable to retain the order of the letters in his mind, and that he was being told to look up spellings in the dictionary but found it all impossible.

Shortly after he had been diagnosed as dyslexic, when he was a little over ten years old, Sylvia sat down with Paul and talked at length about what it was like. Over a period of two weeks, she wrote down, word for word, the following account of Paul's thoughts and observations:

I get muddled up about the time, especially on quiet days at home when nothing in particular is happening. Time doesn't seem to fit in with me and I don't understand the clocks. I think it's lunchtime but it's way before. Then sometimes the day seems to be ahead of me and it has finished before I think it should have done. On days at school there is a set pattern so I know where I am.

Watches muddle me. I forget to look at them and I often read the numbers on a digital watch the wrong way round. Sometimes I mix up 5 and 2 because they both have a curvy shape so I don't always tell the time properly. I can never look at an ordinary clock and just know the time. I have to look carefully to see which is the big hand and which is the little hand, and then count all the five minute sections. I often get it wrong and I never know whether I'm right or not.

I used to get a funny feeling when we had to do reading because I knew that it would be 'Oh Paul . . . really!' again. I knew that everybody would get fed up because I couldn't get it right. It is hard for me to go down from one line to the next because I just seem to lose my place and the words seem to move about in front of my eyes. I might read a word like 'Matthew' at the top of the page and then I read it as 'Michael' when I see it again at the bottom. But I don't know why this happens.

I don't notice the full stops and things because I have to spend all my time thinking about the letters. This happens when I write as well so I just do very long sentences!

I used to like books with pictures in because I could work out the meaning of a story by looking at the pictures. It is hard for me sometimes to understand all the meaning of the story because if the book is difficult I have to use all of my brain just to work out what the words are. I often miss out the little words like 'a' and 'the' but sometimes I put words in that aren't there. I always wanted to read the wrong way across a page and I sometimes read words backwards, but I don't do this so much now.

When I'm writing people often tell me that I have the margin on the wrong side of the paper so that the paper is really upside down, but it doesn't seem wrong to me. I don't write back to front in mirror-writing any more because I'm not allowed to, but it used to be easier for me that way. I would prefer to write the other way across a page. My brain is back to front really.

I find copying the hardest thing of all. It takes me twice as long as it does to write my own story. Copying is really difficult. To everyone else the sentences look only a few centimetres long but to me it is like looking at acres and acres. It is as if the other children have a small area to paint and they do it easily and quickly. But I seem to be facing a massive blank wall that goes on for ever.

I try to get it all to look smooth and nice but I keep missing bits and having to go over it again and again so it never looks good and never gets finished. I can't just look at a word and remember it like everyone else. I can only hold the letters in my mind for a few seconds and even then, when I try to write them down, I get them in the wrong order. I have to keep looking back at the word I am copying and write it one letter at a time which takes ages and I often lose my place.

I remember words by the pattern of the letters. With a word like 'sugar' I remember that it has a flat-topped shape so I know that it hasn't got a tall letter in it and it can't be 'sh' at the beginning although it sounds as though it should be.

I see the outline shapes of words so when I look at a page I see the words as patterns. When I do manage to really learn a word, I throw the shape away and just keep the word in my mind.

When I write stories, my main problem is the spelling and it is hard for me to work out sentences, capital letters and everything. I used to write really good stories but nobody else could read them because I missed out letters, whole lines and full stops. But I didn't know that I'd missed them out.

I could read the stories myself but sometimes I wouldn't be reading them from the paper, I'd be reading them in my mind, my mind filled in the gaps. I have a lot of good stories in my head but I just can't write them down.

Understanding is a problem – working out the different signs. If I look at an '×' I guess, but I'm never really sure whether I should multiply or add. Plus and minus is no problem. What is the sign with the line and two dots? My mind just goes blank and I have to ask.

Plus and minus are easy because I have been doing them for a long time. I'm hoping that the others will stay in my mind soon. I find learning tables very difficult. I have to say a table right through really quickly and if I stop to think of an answer I forget where I am up to and have to start over again.

When things are drawn on the blackboard, such as fractions shown by a picture of a bar of chocolate with squares missing, I have to concentrate hard and count the squares in my head. By the time I have worked it out everyone else has reached the end and I just never seem able to take in all the information. I often have to

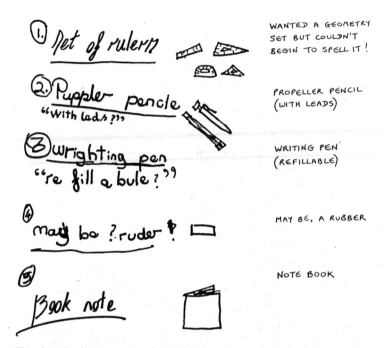

This shopping list was written by Paul Davis when he was ten and three-quarters.

go to my teacher and tell him that I don't understand, because my brain takes things in more slowly. This annoys me.

At school, as the work got harder, I started getting stuck again and again. I couldn't understand why I couldn't do the work when everyone else could. I just wanted to cry and I thought, 'I am thick'. I started to get depressed. I would stand in a queue waiting for my book to be marked, watching all the others getting ticks for their work. It would be my turn and I'd get Xs and be told to redo the work. I would still get Xs and I'd be told that I wasn't trying. So I would have to rewrite the same piece of work several times and I'd make different mistakes each time.

I never knew that I'd done it wrong. It always looked fine to me. Sometimes my work would be put in the bin. I didn't like this but I suppose it looked like rubbish.

I really felt angry at times and I wanted to scream and even hit out but I didn't because I'd end up in trouble and there would be a letter sent home to Mum and Dad and they would be angry with me.

Sometimes I look as though I'm not trying because I just have to stop thinking and look out of the window to give my brain a rest.

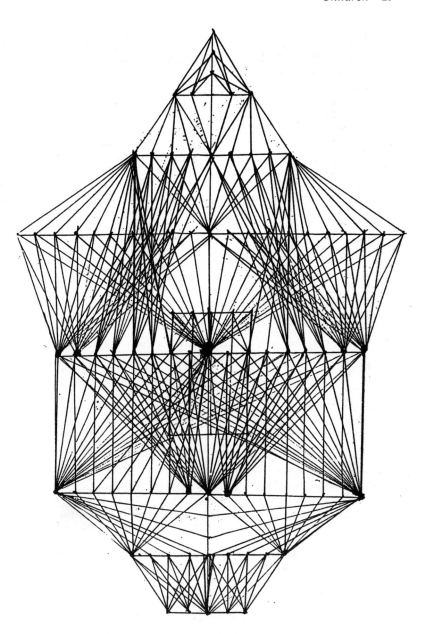

This design was produced by Paul Davis in ten minutes, shortly after he wrote out the shopping list on the previous page.

It's as though I have a battery in my head which is running down, while the other children run on Duracell!

I find it hard to remember all my things . . . spelling book, lunch box, swimming kit, etc. It is always a strain on my mind and I'm nervous until I get home and check what I've got. I often have to go back for something so it's lucky I live near the school.

Other children often make fun of me and call me names. I am picked on a lot and a gang used to set on me because they said I was too thick to do anything about it. I was called 'thicko' and much worse things. But now I have been assessed I tell people that I'm not thick, just dyslexic. What I would really like to do when I am grown up is to help other dyslexics so that they can be happy.

Left and right really don't mean anything to me. I can work out which is my left hand because it's the one I write with, though I still have to think about it. At Cubs I often salute and handshake with the wrong hand. It's just luck if I get it right. I tend to watch the others.

I put a secret Biro mark on the flag rope when nobody was looking so now I know that's the one I pull for the flag to go up. Before that I used to pull the wrong rope. I once pulled the rope very hard and the flag went up instead of down and started to come off its runner. You're not supposed to look at the ropes but the picture of the Queen. I get nervous when it's my turn.

Having problems with left and right makes me feel rather angry because I can't join in properly with everything. In rounders, when I first played, we were told to run 'right' round the bases. I was the first batter and I ran left. I scored a rounder but I scored it the wrong way round, so it wasn't allowed. When friends shout out directions in games, I usually run the wrong way and get caught.

There are a few advantages to being dyslexic. My brain seems to be good at thinking up scientific ideas and building working models. I also like drawing pictures and I quite like making up poems. It's funny that one of my friends is the cleverest boy in the class and he's brilliant at English. He says I'm good at all the things he isn't good at. Together we seem to make one very clever person.

I seem to notice more things than other people. I can tell the make of a car by looking at its hub-caps. I learnt this when I was in a push-chair and could only see at a low level. I remember buildings in detail and especially the roofs and ceilings like in St Paul's. I used to tell Daddy about a big white house with a long drive and it turned out to be a place I was taken to when I was only two years old – before I could talk even.

I don't think that I'll ever have a car because I don't expect that I'll be able to get a good job and earn much money. I always wanted to be an architect but I expect I'll end up as a cleaner. Mr Adams (the educational psychologist) told me I could be a scientist if I wanted to but I shouldn't think I will because I'll always look stupid to people.

I know inside that I'm not stupid, but I look stupid to everyone else because all the things that I *can't* do are the things that you *have* to do at school.

After Paul had been diagnosed as dyslexic his parents successfully fought a battle with their local education authority to have him Statemented. Eventually the LEA agreed to pay for him to attend Grenville College, a school near Bideford in north Devon which has a dyslexia unit attached to it.

Going away from home was difficult and it took Paul about a year to settle down. However, he was in a school where being dyslexic was commonplace and he made a lot of friends. Three years later, when he was fourteen, Sylvia his mother was pleased with the progress he had been able to make: 'We have seen Paul grow in self-confidence and he seems quite excited about choosing his GCSE options,' she said.

He is keenly taking part in the Duke of Edinburgh Award scheme and has started to enjoy sport for the first time, especially basketball, swimming and sailing. What is particularly amazing is to hear him talk animatedly about books. He rang recently to say he had just finished *Of Mice and Men* by John Steinbeck and thought it was brilliant.

He still has a tendency to misread notices but is learning to double-check. He still has an enormous problem with spelling but refuses to let it get him down. He is, of course, fortunate to be where he is with teachers who are fully conscious of his problems and who look at the content of his work rather than at all the errors. He is showing promise with subjects like Craft, Design and Technology and is talking about a career in engineering.

Obviously he has a long way to go, but he is beginning to cope. He took a phone call for me at half-term and I heard him explain to the caller that he was dyslexic and would be grateful if she could speak more slowly to enable him to write the message down. He was not embarrassed to admit he had a problem and he dealt with it in a totally matter-of-fact way. That was an enormous advance.

STEVEN BONFIELD

When Steven Bonfield was ploughing through his A levels perhaps the most significant thing about his day was the beginning. At half past eight every morning a car would draw up outside his house at Bryncethin, near Bridgend in south Wales, and out would step his best friend, John Merrick.

Inside the house John would stand in the hallway checking that Steven had everything he needed for the day – his homework from the night before, bag, games kit, keys, cash. Then together they would head off for their comprehensive school just a few miles away.

The story is revealing for two reasons. First, by the time he was in his middle teens Steven had acquired a close friend. Second, despite having made it through GCSEs and into the sixth form he was still having to cope with his dyslexia, a continual handicap. From the point of view of his parents, however, the fact that he was coping was a kind of miracle.

For at the time his problem was identified, when he was eleven years old, Steven had no friends of his own age, hated school, was bullied, was well behind in reading and spelling, was withdrawn and introverted. Altogether he presented a combination of problems that defeated his parents and teachers alike.

However, after he had been assessed at the Staines Dyslexia Institute the Mid Glamorgan Education Authority finally recognized his problem. As a result Steven's life changed completely. It took five years of struggle, hard work and concentrated, dedicated special teaching. Yet by the end of this time Steven had become an integrated, articulate, cheerful and capable person. In fact, he provides a testimony to what dyslexic children can achieve, even when, as in his case, they are diagnosed relatively late in childhood.

Steven passed five GCSEs with good enough grades to take him into the sixth form to study Maths, Physics and Computer Science; and this despite still having to cope with severe dyslexia which he described at the time in the following matter-of-fact way:

> How would you describe my condition? Well I have a lack of short-term memory. I just can't memorize random sets of numbers. I was sixteen before I knew all the months of the year in order. My times tables are impossible. Well, I suppose I know up to four or five, but sevens, eight and nines are a problem. Division is completely beyond me. I just use a calculator all the time. I go everywhere with a notebook and calculator.
>
> Sometimes I get quite a physical reaction, a kind of nervous reaction, when I read. When I have to read out loud, for instance, my nose will run, my eyes water and occasionally I'll even start to wheeze. Nowadays I'm a lot more confident and actually I can read

very well and normally I'm quite happy about it. But then there's the odd occasion when I'll come across a word I can't read straight away and it'll take me right back. If it's in public, like reading aloud in class and if I haven't rehearsed it, there I'll go again, eyes streaming away.

Mind you I like to read, though it's still an effort and I have to be really interested to keep going more than five minutes. You see I have to read each word individually, sometimes even individual letter by letter.

I go cold every time I see a form. Certain things I know I can't do. I can't remember an address if someone gives it to me or a telephone number. Generally there are people around who can help. It might mean that I have to explain the problem but I don't find that terribly embarrassing. That's not the point. It's just arduous after a while explaining it to the umpteenth person in the same week.

And my spelling, of course, is all over the shop. Copying things down in school is a continual problem. I copy words individually off the board, or out of a book. So I keep losing the place where I am, miss out the words or simply repeat them.

I usually try and avoid doing it, either by borrowing other people's work or by photocopying. When I do copy from the board I seem to have to keep to the lines that are on the blackboard. As a result the lines in my book are all over the place. But that is the only way I can get it down.

If I'm in the middle of taking notes and something else intervenes, perhaps someone asks a question, and my concentration is interrupted, then I easily get lost. Remembering the next sentence when you've looked down from the board is almost impossible when you are three or four sentences behind trying to keep up and trying to listen to someone at the same time. But as I say, I usually avoid taking notes.

I do have to work harder, take more care and take more time than other people. There always seems to be that extra bit you have to do. In the beginning it feels like you're taking two steps back for every one step forward. But gradually you become better at doing things. The difference between you and other people gets less, and if you work at it, gradually you don't have to work that much harder than everyone else.

When you first start you don't see the massive strides that you are making because they are all veiled by other things, I suppose the whole emotional side of it. You are always the last person to see any success.

Dyslexia is a disability like blindness. It's never going to go away. The last person to be convinced I was dyslexic was me. I just thought I was thick at school and that it was my fault. I can remember the anger and frustration I felt, especially earlier on, and I still do I suppose, though not as much. I just felt very uptight all the time. There seemed nothing I could do to improve the situation.

This cool, objective account was made by Steven when he was seventeen years old. What it describes was the result of five years of intensive effort by himself, his teachers and his parents.

When he was small Steven had to be dragged to primary school, often protesting all the way. His father, Geoffrey, a project manager with British Steel, recalled one occasion:

> I didn't often take him to school but I vividly remember taking him once, right through the playground to the door and he was all right until I let go of his hand. Then he seemed to panic and kicked and screamed in a hysterical sort of way. You can imagine how disconcerted I was. This went on for some time until the teacher came out and dragged him away, telling me to leave Steven at the school gate in future.
>
> We were at loss to know what to do about it. We were casting around in the mist really.

Steven had remedial teaching for his reading. His mother, Georgina, a health authority training officer, remembers:

> He did improve a bit but it was so tortuous. He'd bring some reading work home from school and we'd try and read it with him. But it was an impossible exercise. One word he'd read correctly on one line, but it would be wrong on the next. They'd be simple words like *and* and *the*. It was such a misery for him, absolute misery. There was no joy in it, no success for him and as a result it was a kind of nightmare.

When Steven was nine his parents consulted the school's headmaster, who brought in a child psychologist. 'They said that Steven did have a reading problem but that with remedial teaching it would come right,' said his father. 'I remember Georgina asked if the problem could be dyslexia but we were told that the authority didn't recognize it and so, even if it was, it wouldn't make any difference.'

In all the circumstances it was deeply ironic that when Steven was seven he was chosen to be among a small group of children from the school to travel to Castle Howard in North Yorkshire to receive a prize on behalf of his school from Princess Anne for a school spelling competition. The family still have the local newspaper cutting, including his picture and the headline – 'MY WORD! DIDN'T THEY SPELL WELL'. The reason Steven was chosen was because he was one of the brighter, more articulate children. As he recalls, 'Half the class thought I was a dumbo, and half an egghead. When I was ten I was known as the mad professor.'

Georgina added, 'He was a weird child really, almost an adult child. He loved wearing suits and ties, things that other kids didn't wear, and mixing with grown-ups. He had virtually no friends of his own age, but seemed to spend a lot of time with us or just on his own.' Steven said:

> I remember liking books. Mum and Dad spent hours reading to me things like *Lord of the Rings*. I didn't read them myself of course. I liked home and hated school. School was something you did and then you went home.
>
> There were a thousand reasons why I didn't like school. There was the work, and the people, but it was the work mainly. I wanted to work but somehow I just couldn't do it. Eventually I'd sort of turn off and dream my way through the day. Actually, that's quite easy to do if you are undisturbed for long enough. You get almost catatonic. I don't think it helped either because I was always well behaved, very quiet. So no one took any notice. I suppose I was happily glossed over and ignored, which made everyone's life easier.
>
> When I got home I used to dread the next day coming. The next day at school crept nearer and nearer until eventually I was thinking about it all the time. Even the weekend would be the same. Saturday would be OK but then by the time Sunday morning came round I'd start thinking there'd be school on Monday.

In his last year at primary school Steven's parents became very worried and, in desperation, sought help from their local Citizens Advice Bureau. They were directed to the Staines Dyslexia Institute where Steven was found to be dyslexic. Armed with this evidence Steven's parents persuaded Mid Glamorgan Education Authority to make a Statement concerning his special needs, the first one it had made in relation to dyslexia. From then on Steven's prospects changed dramatically.

As soon as he entered secondary school he began having one-to-one help from a series of teachers trained in special needs and helping dyslexic children. With one-to-one help, nine hours a week, Steven made rapid progress during his first year at comprehensive school. At the start of the year the school had suggested he should be placed in the remedial section of the class. By the end he had moved into the top-class A stream.

In his second year, however, his progress faltered. His special needs teacher at the time, Elizabeth Richards, recalled:

Steven was a contradictory character. He obviously had great potential and intellectually he was very able. But he lacked the tools which would give him the freedom to use his intelligence in the written word, and he desperately wanted to write. When I first met him he was twelve with a reading age of nine, and a spelling age of seven. By the time he was fourteen his reading age had pulled up, almost to his chronological age, and his spelling age had reached about nine and a half.

At twelve years old he was aloof, rather cold and unforthcoming about his difficulties. He tended to keep everything inside himself. He knew he had a lot to give but he was unable to warm to individuals and found it difficult to communicate.

Steven himself remembers the time well. 'I felt a kind of hatred for the world,' he said.

Things had been going quite well in my first year. I had improved a bit, but suddenly all the changes began to throw me. I suppose I was reaching the age where hormones start jumping, where adolescence kicks in. I seemed to reach one of those natural plateaux on the learning curve which interlocked with general unhappiness in other parts of my life.

Towards the end of the autumn term Elizabeth Richards spotted Steven one day by himself in the playground. 'I was able to observe him from a distance and he was without a friend,' she said.

He was completely alone, standing very close to a large stone wall which ringed the playground area and I just had an awful feeling inside that something was badly wrong.

I'd sensed that things were difficult and that he was finding it hard to cope. Success wasn't coming quickly enough for him. The skills he was learning with me were not being transferred to the mainstream classroom situation. Steven wanted things to happen far more quickly than they were actually able to and I think he also resented me intruding into his life.

Steven vividly recalled how matters came to a head.

She was telling me off for not doing something and I suddenly shouted back at her. It was a watershed moment. I'd been shouting about things at home too, so I suppose I was generally difficult.

But Mrs Richards was very good. We began talking things through a lot. That was a turning point for me, I think. From being nowhere and facing a bleak future, I began somehow to feel good about things in a way that had not happened before.

Elizabeth Richards described how she dealt with the aftermath of this confrontation.

I alerted the other people who were concerned with Steven's well-being, the head of the school, the psychologist and the advisory service and, of course, Steven's parents. We met very quickly the following week to discuss his problems and from then on we were more conscious that we had to help him as a person rather than just concentrating on raising his reading and spelling ages.

It became more a matter of concern to help him get over his crisis of personality and his difficulties within himself than it was actually to teach him to read and write. That would come later, but only when we had him as a happy and stable individual.

So from then on we refocused the teaching. It became more a counselling exercise, more a matter of raising his self-esteem, of increasing his motivation and providing him with strategies for coping with his problems.

It seemed to me that the events from the past had not been resolved in his mind and they were, in fact, making him very unhappy in the present. I believe actually that he was very bitter about his past experiences.

Steven agreed. 'I was certainly frustrated with the world and all its workings, without any question,' he said.

I felt I'd been hard done by in every respect, socially and educationally. Although people had been trying to help me, for a year at least, it still hadn't really filtered through. I was frustrated, too, about my inability to make any friends, which I think was the main thing.

Social things are always the ones that bite, that make you depressed. You don't get depressed because you can't do the work even though that's an underlying factor. You're depressed really because you've got no one to talk to.

It was hard talking things out, certainly for the first three or four sessions. But after a while I began saying and revealing things I'd never let out before. I started to challenge myself and things around me in a way I had never done, verbally at least. I suppose it was a kind of self-analysis.

Elizabeth Richards added:

As I saw it, it was my function to help Steven achieve a degree of self-realization and so come to terms with his difficulties. He had to recognize what his problems were, what was worrying him, and how he was going to cope in the classroom. He was very sensitive and vulnerable to criticism. He had to cope with the fact that he couldn't achieve what he felt he ought to be achieving.

Then he had to go out into the playground which was a nightmare for him because he had no friends. He had to survive playtime and lunchtime. So he needed precise coping strategies for those situations.

Then we began looking at what was underlying his problems, examining the past and discovering what had gone wrong. In many ways I think he had been a victim of his lack of social skills. He had been from a small boy a very isolated child. He always felt, I believe, that he was different and that it was difficult for him to come to terms with himself and to relate to other people. In school he had always been placed according to his actual attainment level, which was well below his real intellectual level. So he was totally out of touch with other children both in the classroom and in the playground. He had to evolve strategies for how he was going to reach out and make contact with his peers. He had to learn how to make friends.

The process proved very successful. At the end of his second year Steven moved up a stream. There he found a circle of friends, in particular John Merrick. Another breakthrough came when he was the only pupil in the school to win a distinction in a drama examination. This entailed acting and reading aloud. 'It was the first real success he had had and it gave him recognition amongst the rest of the school, staff and children,' said Elizabeth Richards. 'I think that was a kind of jumping-off point for Steven.'

The point must be made that it is exceptional for a pupil, even with Steven's difficulties, to receive so much help inside the state system. For an extended period he was receiving one-to-one help for a total of nine hours a week – thirteen periods across two and a half days. Steven was fortunate because he was the first child to be Statemented for dyslexia by his local education authority. As a result he became in effect a test case for an LEA feeling its way. The time, empathy and attention that were given to Steven are not, by any means, universal. 'The time allocation was without doubt generous,' said Elizabeth Richards. 'But it certainly paid off and shows, I think, what can be achieved.'

Steven himself has no doubts that without the support he received he would not have pulled through. 'I think I would have thrown myself over a cliff,' he said.

It was that bad. I was getting desperate. At the very least I'd be sweeping roads. I certainly wouldn't have got into the sixth form. Passing sufficient GCSEs was important of course but it wasn't the main achievement for me. The goal I think I reached was that I became happy with myself. I was able to consider myself normal, though I hesitate to use that word.

RACHEL JONES

A reading of this book might lead those unfamiliar with dyslexic people to conclude that at least they are not short of words to say, even if they find them difficult to read, write and spell. But while it is true that many dyslexics are highly articulate, many are not. More generally, it is often the case that they simply prefer to be quiet and blend into the background, rather than become too noticeable.

Rachel Jones is a good example. A quiet, shy girl, she none the less gives the impression of being fully aware of what is going on, but from behind a mask of apparent non-involvement. Rachel's experience is typical in many other respects as well. She falls into the majority group of dyslexic children who, on that spectrum of mild to severe, are moderately affected.

Then again, her problems were only identified after a long and insistent struggle by her parents. They have been recognized by her local education authority, which nevertheless has refused to use the label 'dyslexia'. Its advisers preferred to use the catch-all phrase 'specific learning difficulty'. And despite a Statement of Rachel's special education needs at last being agreed when she was ten years old, these needs met incomprehension and lack of understanding at her school.

Rachel's parents – her father is a general practitioner and her mother a nurse – sensed there was something unusual about her progress when she was very young, between four and five years old. 'From the beginning we knew Rachel had problems,' said her mother, Caroline. 'She didn't want to go to school, often complained of tummy ache, was disruptive in class, liked drawing but hated books, and she tired very easily.'

When she was six Rachel was assessed by an independent educational psychologist who concluded that she was of above average intelligence (114 on the pre-school scale) and probably dyslexic though it was too early to say conclusively. Definitely, however, she needed special help.

Rachel was taught by a remedial teacher at school, and for a while by another remedial teacher at home for an hour a week. However, these teachers were not trained in techniques appropriate for teaching dyslexic children and little progress was made. 'I remember one of the remedial teachers saying to me that she simply couldn't work out how to teach Rachel,' said Caroline.

When she was seven her parents moved her to another primary school near her home where they discerned that the teachers would be more accommodating in dealing with her problems. 'They tended to concentrate on what she was good at rather than what she was continually failing to achieve,' said Caroline. However, she was still not receiving the specialist help that dyslexic children need.

Long negotiations began with the local education authority for a Statement of Needs to be made. Meanwhile Rachel's parents arranged for her to be taken out of school once a week for three-quarters of an hour and taught privately by a teacher trained in dyslexia techniques. For the first time Rachel began to get on top of her problems and make some progress.

The LEA offered to provide this help in school, from a remedial teacher. Her parents insisted, however, that if this was to be done it had to be with a teacher trained in dyslexia techniques. The LEA replied that the remedial teacher was appropriately qualified. There was an impasse.

Meetings were held between Rachel's parents, the school's headmistress and LEA advisers including an educational psychologist. Rachel's parents were armed with further reports from their independent educational psychologist, indicating that although chronologically nearly ten years old, Rachel had a reading age of only six and a half. He recommended that she should be Statemented and provided with the appropriate help. Eventually, a year later, just as Rachel was poised to enter secondary school, a Statement was issued in the following terms:

> *Rachel is a girl of average intelligence who is experiencing problems with reading, spelling and writing resulting from specific learning difficulties. She needs an individually designed programme aimed at developing visual and auditory memory skills and which is based on a phonic approach to reading. Such a programme would aim to improve auditory and visual sequencing, sound blending and whole word recognition.*

The provision to meet these Statemented needs was defined as:

> *Placement in mainstream class with regular support and supervision of an individually designed programme, provided by a specialist teacher of children with specific learning difficulties, as 90 minutes' help delivered in three 30 minute sessions.*

What this meant in practice, during Rachel's first term in secondary school, was removal from normal lessons three times a week to be taught on a one-to-one basis by a remedial teacher versed in dyslexia techniques. Despite this it did not provide an adequate answer. 'I find the special lessons boring and I don't like leaving my class,' Rachel said.

> What we do is basic and very simple. Anyway, the time we spend actually working is not very much. It takes me five minutes to reach where we have the special lesson, and another five minutes to return to the class. We just chat generally for another five minutes as well. It's really a bit of a waste of time.

At a parents' evening at the end of her first term Rachel's mother and father discovered that most of her teachers were unaware that a Statement of Special Needs had been made. Some teachers expressed puzzlement at her lack of progress and sometimes erratic standards. Others complained that her work was untidy and her spelling odd. Her Maths teacher confessed he couldn't understand how she often produced excellent work in class, but then failed completely in tests.

It was only after they had seen the headteacher for a second time that Rachel's parents felt satisfied that the message about her problems had been passed on to the teachers generally. However, they became worried when some months later they were told that Rachel would undoubtedly have more problems when she went into the second year. There the work would become more demanding and it was possible that she would have to be put down a set and receive some remedial help.

'If I go down a set it will be boring and everyone will start talking about me as thick all over again,' Rachel said. Faced with this prospect Rachel's parents determined that they would remove her from the state system and send her away to be taught privately, at a school dedicated to helping dyslexic children. They had one in mind, where Rachel had already attended a summer course. 'I liked it there,' Rachel said. 'The teachers didn't seem like teachers. They treated you as though you were a normal person. I don't want to go away to school and be away from home and away from my friends. But it would be worse to be put down a set and have everybody think I was stupid again.'

EARLY IDENTIFICATION

All the experts are agreed that the earlier a child is identified as dyslexic the better he or she can be helped through school. This points to the need for all children who exhibit early reading difficulties to be screened for dyslexia as soon as possible, certainly around the ages of six or seven. There is a strong case for screening all children of this age who are placed in the remedial section of their class.

Such screening should not simply be aimed at identifying reading ability. As Professor Tim Miles has pointed out, this will necessarily reveal only an amorphous mass of poor readers of all kinds. In his book *Understanding Dyslexia* he noted:

> Although this group may well contain children who are dyslexic, many of the brighter dyslexic children may escape this particular net, since their reading age may not be all that far behind the norm for their age, their relative weakness being masked by their high intelligence. Such children may, of course, be very unhappy in school if suitable provision is not made for them.

Children with dyslexia can usually be distinguished from those with, for instance, a mild mental handicap by their skills and obvious intelligence in other areas. A child of between five and six might come across as an intelligent, able conversationalist but at the same time be unable to write his or her name, copy letters or shapes with a pencil or bricks, cope with buttons, bows and other fine motor tasks. Alternatively, a child may be able to copy shapes but be unable to repeat numbers, be clumsy and lack co-ordination, and generally be a late speech developer. All these are indications of dyslexia, especially if coupled with a family background of literacy difficulties.

Given that by overwhelming expert consent dyslexia is a genetically inherited condition, it should be possible to identify it in children before they reach school age. Finding reliable ways of achieving this was one of the objectives of a five-year research project begun at the Medical Research Council's Cognitive Development Unit in London in 1993. Focusing on children in families where one or both adults are dyslexic, it aims to produce early indicators of children at risk of developing dyslexia.

Dr Uta Frith, the senior scientist in charge of the project, said:

If we believe that dyslexia has genetic causes, it is not a wild guess to assume that it will produce manifestations in the pre-school years. Eventually, we hope to produce a means of making a diagnosis before a child fails at school. The aim is to avoid the unnecessary problems and repercussions on a child's self-esteem of being seen as a failure before remedial action is taken.

Possible indicators are already widely appreciated and begin, of course, with a family history of literacy difficulties and delay in speech development. Then again, a pre-school child may show a delay in the development of speech and language; may seem to be developing normally in most areas but have a marked difficulty in copying shapes with a pencil or with bricks; may have difficulty with sequencing, such as coloured bead and brick patterns or sequential pictures; and may have difficulty remembering the order of simple instructions. In addition to these difficulties, a child may show signs of clumsiness, poor co-ordination, easy distractibility and poor concentration.

Such indicators are, of course, only indicators and a matter for what is inevitably subjective observation. None the less, the more parents are aware of potential problems the greater the likelihood that dyslexic children can have the benefit of an early identification of their condition. Only then will the worst threats of all to dyslexic children – feelings of failure, guilt and low self-esteem – be lifted before they have time to take hold.

Chapter 3

Adults

So much attention has been given to the needs of dyslexic children, to arguments about provision in the schools, the role of parents, teachers and local education authorities, that it is all too easily forgotten that there are many thousands of adult dyslexics for whom much of this is irrelevant.

At least today dyslexia, if still a subject of dispute and controversy, is a topical issue about which knowledge is rapidly spreading. Yet only a few years ago this was simply not the case. For many years there will be adult dyslexics who will never discover the root cause of problems they have been unable to articulate. Others, probably fewer but more fortunate, will discover late in life and often by accident that there is an explanation for their being marked out as different which is not based on some humiliating inadequacy.

It is worth giving attention to the experiences of such people, not only for what they tell us about dyslexia as such, but also to encourage other adults to ask themselves whether they might be dyslexic.

The adult experience of dyslexia, certainly as relayed in these pages, provides a salutary warning of what can happen to children who fail to be recognized as dyslexic early in their life. The pain, misery and frustration so amply testified in this chapter is one dimension. Another is the underlying consequences for society as a whole. Typically, as has been said, dyslexic people are of at least average and often above average intelligence. When this is added to the inevitable humiliation and frustration of dyslexia and then mixed with misunderstanding and maltreatment at school and sometimes even in the home, the potential for deviant behaviour is very high. Evidence pointing to the harsh possibility that up to half of Britain's prison population may be dyslexic to some degree will be surveyed in the final chapter.

This is not to say, of course, that dyslexia is inevitably linked with deviant behaviour and crime. However, the potential is certainly there. As Krysia Martin, a teacher in the Education Department at Pentonville Prison in London put it:

> It would be too simplistic to suggest that dyslexia alone is responsible for offending behaviour, but certainly the feelings of inadequacy, low self-esteem from not being able to read and write, and the feeling of not being heard or understood does not help. Although I have done no specific survey of dyslexia in prison, it is clear that a very high proportion of men who ask for help with literacy problems are dyslexic.

As it is, the main work and studies of adult dyslexia so far undertaken have been with students who present themselves with literacy problems in higher and further education. What these have shown is that adult dyslexics have very different problems, and require very different solutions, as compared with those who are fortunate enough to be recognized at an earlier age in school.

No one is more familiar with what is required than Cynthia Klein, director of the Language and Literacy Unit at London's Southwark College. 'The dyslexic adult invariably comes with very specific needs,' she said. 'As one colleague who is used to teaching children put it, dyslexic adults want exactly what they want, when they want it – right now!'

She gave as an example a person who might be in a job that involves writing reports, which that person is unable to do. Another might have been offered promotion but feels unable to take it on because it will mean having to write. Someone else might want to re-enter education but is frustrated by the lack of minimal education requirements. 'Adult dyslexics often need practical "life" strategies, as most of them say their biggest problem is other people,' Cynthia Klein said. 'Students in work situations need to know how to explain their difficulties to alleviate confusions and anxieties about their performance, to develop specific practical aids to minimize difficulties, and to ask for the support they need.'

Dyslexic people are often highly articulate. That does not mean, however, that they can always readily communicate exactly what a problem is or explain precisely why it is they have failed to understand something. Cynthia Klein described the following case.

> A student doing silversmithing had been told that she had not developed her design adequately. Although she asked her tutor what he meant, she didn't understand his answer and didn't dare ask again. She asked her fellow students but didn't understand their explanations either.
>
> I suggested she ask him to show her an example of how to develop a design. Her eyes lit up. She hadn't thought of that. I think that's a good example of how dyslexics get 'trapped' in abstract language and need a way out into something more concrete.

Another example was a Social Studies student on a practical placement who was asked by her supervisor to explain the theoretical basis of her decisions in a particular case. 'As she didn't know what the supervisor meant she merely appeared not to know her material,' said Cynthia Klein. 'In fact, she needed to learn how to say, "I don't understand what you mean when you ask that question. Can you put it another way or give me an example?" '

To survive, adult dyslexics find myriad means to circumvent problems. Generally these entail simply avoiding the written word, for instance paying by cash rather than writing a cheque. Often, however, they can be highly ingenious in overcoming their difficulties. Cynthia Klein said she had several students who had learnt the alphabet by singing it. Another student managed to pass his exams by using an ancient Roman mnemonic trick. He visualized all the formulae he had to remember on different places in the examination room and when he entered the room they all came flooding back.

She encourages students to use 'right brain' strategies which many may have already discovered but not adapted to learning situations. An example is a student who remembered phone numbers by tapping them on a push button phone. Would he be able to use the same approach by learning to spell on a keyboard? 'Many students do find their spelling improves on word processors – and not just because of a spellcheck,' Cynthia Klein said. 'One student we had felt he could write and spell better on a word processor simply because he was using both hands.'

Not many dyslexic adults have the benefit of such advice, however. The following accounts of the experiences of people who have discovered they were dyslexic at different stages in their adult life show that while their stories contrast markedly they have certain things in common. All are profoundly glad to have identified themselves as dyslexic. At last they now have a rational explanation for what had hitherto seemed arbitrary problems for which they were to blame. All have been remarkably resourceful in coping with the problems they have faced. And while the severity of their experiences varies widely – sometimes reflecting their circumstances as children, sometimes sheer luck – all wished they had known they were dyslexic much, much earlier.

JOANNE COOK

In her mid-twenties Joanne Cook comes over on the face of it as a bright, fluent person, in every sense a controlled and integrated personality. And, indeed, that is what she self-consciously wants and tries to be. 'I know I'm getting there,' she will say.

Yet not far beneath her cheerful exterior is a jumble of emotions and feelings only now, late in the day, being discovered, addressed and understood. For Joanne has struggled, for most of her life unknowingly, with acute dyslexia, compounded by severe and related myopia.

Most of what such a person requires – support, understanding and emotional stability – has been denied Joanne at many stages of her life. Only when she was twenty-four years old was her condition identified. By then she had experienced an enormous amount of damage, pain and frustration. Despite this she has emerged, if not unscathed, certainly mature beyond her years. 'I know that I'm intelligent, good with my hands, a creative person,' she said. 'I have these qualities and they are precious to me. As a kid I was told I was stupid and thick and I was pretty scared a lot of the time. I still am. But still I am, I think, a caring and sympathetic person. I could be quite different, you know, given what I've been through.'

Joanne was born in Cheltenham in 1967. Her mother was a secretary, her father a builder whose work meant he had to move around a good deal. That presented an immediate problem for

Joanne since she was constantly changing homes and schools, an acutely disorientating experience for dyslexics. 'I remember I was about six when I began to feel things weren't right, though I couldn't grasp what was the problem,' she said.

> We moved to Evesham and in my new school I was put in a class a year below my age, because I was falling behind I suppose.
>
> That was when my eye problems began too. I should have had glasses. It's a form of double vision and problems with co-ordinating the movements of your eyes. When normal people would unconsciously move their eyes to track, say, words across a page, I would move my head. Sometimes you feel the world is spinning round and you can't catch up.
>
> I think they sensed there was something wrong with my eyes because they put me at the front of the class, but that didn't help. The way we were taught at school involved a lot of reading out of books and copying off the board, which meant I couldn't understand what was going on.
>
> So I just used to sit there and sort of dream and look out of the window. Then when the exams and reports came around there were comments like 'Jo's not concentrating' and things like that.
>
> It just got worse and worse. Every time I went to a different school or into different lessons it was the same way. Nothing was interesting to me. I became withdrawn and bored and sort of put my mind on hold. I felt very isolated and alone.
>
> I suppose I messed about a good bit, became moody and frustrated. Finally we moved back to Cheltenham and I was put in the remedial class of my new school, which was probably the best thing, because at least I could understand a bit more. But no one ever looked at me; for instance I never saw a child psychologist.

When she was fourteen Joanne's parents split up, her father packed his bags and left, and she stayed with her mother in Cheltenham. Though it was unsettling, she says it was probably the best thing for her, in the short-run at least, because of the stormy relationship she had with her father.

> I had an elder brother who did well at school and college and I think dad thought I was just lazy. He'd tell me that I should concentrate.
>
> He did organize some extra lessons for me, in English and Maths, after school. But that was the worst time, you know, when I was tired. And I was just taught parrot fashion. I felt pressured and none of it sank in. And with everybody calling me stupid, at home and in school, well I began to think that maybe I was. So I just stumbled through the education system really.
>
> Mind you I was a bit of a joker and I made friends quite easily. I found ways of working round things. If, for instance, we had

some writing for homework I'd just put it in my bag, take it home
and forget about it. Some things I quite liked – cookery, science,
woodwork – things you could do with your hands. But the big problem I've always had is taking in information, storing it and then
recalling it.

Joanne went into the sixth form, but left halfway through the
first year. 'Leaving was a relief. It was good to be getting into what
I thought was life. But I didn't have a clue what I was going to
do.' She was unemployed for a while, doing odd cleaning and
nursery care cash-in-hand jobs. 'Then I had a stroke of luck,' she
said.

I saw an advertisement for a Youth Training Scheme in Cheltenham
as an industrial weaver. It meant I could start on something without
any qualifications and learn a trade on the job, which was great. It
was something I found I could do, though I took twice as long as
anyone else to fully train, about two years.

The job entailed weaving copper wire and fibreglass thread to
make heated pad elements, used for making aeroplane wings and
propellers. Joanne came to an arrangement where she could work
at home, producing so many units a week. 'It was perfect for
me,' she said. 'I could work at my own time and pace. I felt I was.
achieving something. For the first time I was doing something
entirely by myself.'

At the end of four years, however, she fell out with her supervisor, and left the job. 'I remember the manager came running
down the street after me, pleading with me not to go,' she laughed.
Soon she found another job, as a trainee kiln loader with an
industrial pottery near Gloucester. But this didn't work out as
well. It was heavy work and Joanne found it difficult keeping up
with the pace. 'Things all started going wrong,' she said.

I couldn't cope with the job, which made me tired and frustrated.
I contracted bronchitis from the fumes. I split up with my boyfriend
at the same time. And in the end I had what I think amounted to
a nervous breakdown. That was one of those periods in my life when
I felt totally desperate. I didn't know what to do. I was frightened,
frightened of going for a job interview, frightened of filling in an
application form, frightened of facing up to another job, another
place, more people where I was going to find things difficult, with
people not understanding, not knowing.

Joanne decided on a complete break and responded to an advertisement in a magazine seeking people to live and work on an organic smallholding near Chester. Her time there lasted six months, living in what amounted to a commune. One of the few positive results to come out of this episode was that she made contact with a nearby family where another member of the commune was doing gardening work. 'There were four children in the family, all boys, and three of them were dyslexic,' she said. 'I began to suspect that I might be as well and the mother urged me to be tested. But I was afraid, you know. What if I was tested and they told me there was nothing wrong. Would I be classed as subnormal?'

In any event Joanne became ill again, another relationship ended, and she returned to Cheltenham, but determined now to find out the full extent of her problems. She contacted the local dyslexia association and formed a strong relationship with one of its voluntary workers. She found she could be tested for dyslexia through the local employment office and at last was positively identified.

'It was a relief to know at last that I wasn't making this whole thing up,' she said. 'But to tell the truth I've had difficulty accepting it as well. Obviously I wish I was just an ordinary person. I'm angry and bitter, too, that it was never found out earlier. It's nobody's fault, I suppose, but you do feel let down.'

Joanne is also, at last, being treated for her eye problems. 'I've got two sets of glasses now, one for distance viewing and one for reading,' she said. 'But it's difficult to adjust. It's as though you've grown used to living with a couple of wires crossed and now you have to operate with them straightened up.'

Joanne attended another training scheme, this time furniture restoring, but after six months gave it up. 'The people were great and I learnt a lot, but I just couldn't keep up,' she said.

I became continually frustrated and stressed. I need to find a job where I can use my body and mind together at their own pace, something slow and time-consuming.

But the world doesn't seem to cater for people with my kind of problem. And it's so difficult to explain. Things are twice as hard, take twice as long as for most people. Sometimes I feel as though I want to unzip round the top of my head, take out my brain, and give it a good wash.

In a way it's like living in a maze. Some days are better than others. Some days it's no big problem. Then other days everything comes out backwards, all over the place. If there's a lot going on, then for some unknown reason it's difficult to put things in order in your mind. You just tinker around and end up telling yourself you just don't understand whatever it is you're trying to do. The more you sit and look at it the more you get angry and frustrated and create more of a block in your mind.

All you can do then is just let go and tell yourself you'll deal with it the next day or the day after. But the thing is you mustn't give up. Because there are people out there willing to help and give advice on where to go and what to do. If you feel inside yourself that you want to achieve something then you can do it. You've got to remember that you have qualities that are special to you. I would like to say to people who are frightened of going to get help, and don't know what it might be, you're not the only one.

Don't put yourself up against other people – that's the worst possible thing you can do. If you see somebody doing something so well it's unbelievable, don't put yourself against that person. You're unique to yourself. You are a special person. Do things in your own time and in your own way.

I'm determined inside that I'm going to achieve something. I've met some good people who've helped me and put me in the right direction. But I still don't know what I'm going to do. I've never really had a choice. It's always been taken away.

COLIN NEW

Colin New found his whole life illuminated by finding out, when he was thirty-seven, that he was dyslexic. The discovery came in the course of yet another struggle against adversity that ended in disappointment: examinations for promotion. This is how he remembers the moment:

> The man interviewing me was studying intently the paper I had written. Then he looked up and said, 'Do you mind if I ask you a personal question? Have you ever considered you might be dyslexic?' I was completely thrown. I had never heard the term and was confused by it. So I answered, 'No, I'm a Catholic!'
>
> The man guessed I was dyslexic because he has a dyslexic son and my writing looked similar, getting my bs and ds mixed up, for instance. In one of my examination papers I had written 'dad' for 'bad'. So I had put down something like, 'I feel it would be dad to pursue this course at this time.'

Colin New is a senior prison officer formerly working at Full Sutton High Security Prison near York, but now based in East

Anglia. He had been in the prison service for five years before he took the exams to become a senior officer. He scraped through with difficulty after failing twice, spending night after night writing out essays and having them checked by his wife, Sheila.

Eventually, however, he was spotted as leadership material and urged to apply for the prison service's accelerated promotion scheme. So he entered for exams that led towards a governorship. They entail taking a series of tests that last over a three-day period. It was during his second attempt to pass them that he heard the first hint that he might be dyslexic.

Colin was brought up in Berwick-upon-Tweed and went to school there in the 1950s. Looking back at the period he feels it was a waste of time. 'The gratifying thing about discovering I was dyslexic was that I had to take an extensive range of tests and these proved that I actually have an above average intelligence,' he said. 'Had I known that at school, and had my teachers and parents known it, and had the way I had been taught been adjusted accordingly, then there is no doubt I would have achieved a great deal more than I did.'

As it is, one of his main memories of school is of the inkwells being on the right and his being left-handed, though his teachers insisted he write with his right hand. 'One teacher in particular was adamant that there was no way I was going to write with my left hand,' he said.

> It was totally immoral for me to write with my left hand. Every time she found me secretly having a go with my left hand I got this smacker in the earhole. I kept being told, and I concluded quite rapidly myself, that I was thick and going to lean on a shovel for the rest of my life.
>
> One very hurtful incident often comes to mind. We were doing a history project which I was really interested in and I spent a good two and a half hours at home laboriously writing it all out. Next morning I handed it in, in front of the whole class, and the teacher took one look at it, screwed it up and threw it in the bin. 'If that's the best you can do then don't expect me to mark it,' she said.
>
> You can imagine how angry, frustrated and humiliated I felt. I didn't know what was wrong. Nobody told me there was anything wrong. I was just told I was lazy or stupid or both.

Inevitably he failed the eleven-plus examination. 'I was crying my eyes out,' he recalled.

My mother said she knew I could do it, if I really tried. I knew I had the answers. I just wasn't able to put them down. I became very verbal. Often my mind would work quicker than I was able to talk even. I sometimes found myself saying something, realized I had got ahead of myself, and then landed in a muddle. In the end my confidence was totally destroyed.

Because he was tall he held his own as far as bullying was concerned. 'The kids used to leave me pretty much alone,' he said.

I built up this sense of humour and the teachers referred to me as the class joker. I used to say things and end up in the corridor. The other kids thought that was great. In a way I played a role that was created for me. One of the teachers actually wrote in a report that if I didn't drastically change my attitude I could well end up in prison. Looking back I always have a laugh at that one.

Colin left school at sixteen and after a few years managed to gain a place with the prison service. 'In the entrance exam I scored high enough in the intelligence, maths and general knowledge tests to enable me to scrape in, despite failing the English test,' he said. He managed much of the written work involved in the job, reports and so on, by writing them in rough and getting his wife Sheila to copy them out neatly in good English.

After his dyslexia was diagnosed he was allowed time off work for two years to take special lessons at the Harrogate Dyslexia Institute. At the end of this course he put in for the accelerated promotion exams for a third time, which none the less he failed again. 'The most disconcerting part of the whole three-day affair was the exchange I had with this very eminent lady, who must have been informed by then that I was dyslexic but didn't seem able to take it on board,' he recalled.

She kept saying to me that if I was bright enough to have made it to the interview, I was bright enough to have qualifications. Why hadn't I got them? 'Because I'm dyslexic and I've only just found out,' I answered. They conceded that my written work had improved but all she could harp on about was the absence of any written qualifications – O levels, A levels, degrees. I hadn't got them because I was dyslexic and had never been diagnosed. But I think, you know, she must have just looked at that word on my application form and thought it was my religion.

CHARLIE PAUL

Charlie Paul, now in his early thirties, is a rare example of a person who sailed through his early years largely oblivious of his dyslexic condition and relatively unaffected. He is even able to say that being dyslexic has helped him in his chosen career, as a television and film animator, since it has enabled him to bring a highly original approach to his work.

All this, however, has been the result of a combination of fortunate and highly unusual circumstances. To begin with Charlie comes from a well-off background, with parents who were able to afford to send him to a fee-paying private school, King Alfred's in Golders Green, London. This is a relatively small, mixed day school with some 700 pupils from infants through to sixth form. It has a relaxed, informal atmosphere, with the emphasis placed on personal development as much as examination achievement.

'I don't remember having to take any exams until I was fifteen,' Charlie recalled.

> It was a very gentle education, in fact. The school promoted social skills, relating to people, and gave kids their head in things they were good at and, most importantly for me, at their own pace.
>
> Verbally I could express myself well, but in written work and exams I was terrible. There was a lot of emphasis on project work, for instance in sciences, and I did quite well in that, but when it came to mock O level exams when I was fifteen I failed. Up to then, though it was recognized I was hopeless at spelling, it never seemed a problem.
>
> Perhaps in a way this relaxed attitude was a bad thing since, because I was generally getting on OK, it was never identified as a major problem. As a result it was never really faced up to and diagnosed. On the other hand I enjoyed school, so what's best? And I actually got some O levels, in Art and Geography. Both were subjects where the accent was on the visual. So I went into first-year sixth form and retook Biology, which I passed, though with a pretty low grade.
>
> Looking back, the main reason that I got even those three subjects, apart from them all being related to graphics, was my friendship with Matthew Freeman, son of John Freeman, the broadcaster and diplomat. Matthew was typical of the kind of kids that were at the school, children of famous people with good connections. Anyway he was brilliant. In fact he's now a Harvard professor. He helped me all through school. It was a kind of informal support which I suppose should have come more formally, from the

teachers, if they had realized the extent of my problems. But then I didn't appreciate fully what they were myself.

I wanted to go to art college, but it was obvious I wasn't going to pass any A levels, so I left after one year in the sixth form.

After leaving school Charlie drifted for a couple of years. He worked as a roadie with a rhythm and blues band, travelling around Britain and the United States. Then, through family connections, Charlie found a job with a London firm called Fifth Column which specializes in making tee shirts. This was an important break since it allowed him to move into art work, what he had always wanted to do, drawing designs. These enabled him to build up a portfolio of work which he was able to use to win a place at London's Byam Shaw Art School. It accepted him on the basis of his work rather than the English and Applied Science A levels it normally demanded.

By now Charlie was twenty-six and so, at that time in the mid-1980s, was able to obtain a full grant from his local authority to support him through the three-year diploma course. 'I was dreadful at the essays and in fact I failed my written assessment,' Charlie said. 'But I got through on the basis of my painting work and my enthusiasm for complementary studies.'

He passed the diploma and afterwards fell on his feet again. During the last few weeks of his studies he entered a BBC competition for students – drawing ten pictures for a thirty-second animated sequence – which he won. This was enough to give him an opening into the London world of animation and Harry Films, a company owned by the brother of the man who previously employed him at the Fifth Column tee-shirt company. 'I was brought up in a world where there are many business connections and contacts so in that sense I was extremely fortunate,' Charlie said.

Harry Films specializes in animated sequences for commercials and campaigning organizations, a medium well suited to Charlie's skill. 'The whole approach to the work we do is based on feeling and intuition,' he said. 'Scripts have to follow the images.'

Because he is dyslexic Charlie has developed a highly unusual way of working. Normally animators build up their images by drawing linear sequences, each picture varying slightly, so that when they are filmed frame by frame and run through a projector at speed they give the impression of movement. Charlie achieves the same effect, but in a completely different way. He draws an image, photographs it, and then works another image on top of the one he has already made, photographs that and so on until he has a completed sequence.

> This way of working has given my animation a very distinctive style. Probably my method is unique. I work with large brush strokes and very fast. It seems to me that the process has evolved quite naturally out of the way I think. When you're dyslexic you grab things as you go along. You develop things in a step-ladder kind of way. Somehow that makes things more solid.
>
> It's the only way I can work, at any rate. I couldn't order a story as separate scenes. I have to have a sense of the entire sequence of images, the whole movement, and I have to be able to draw it whole. It's the same with words on a page. Letters by themselves don't make much sense to me, but I can cope with a word as a whole. And it's the same with combinations of images.
>
> It's important for me to see the whole pattern and draw it like that. Then it's as though I'm using my own language which is coming from inside myself. When I can work like that it doesn't frighten me. It makes me feel that I have everything under control.

Charlie says it was always his dream to be able to divorce art from the written and spoken word, a dream he began to define when he was at art school. 'Animation work in my style is perfect for that,' he said.

> I've always wanted to make images that in a way are pure as images, uncluttered by any verbal references.
>
> I suppose that's a direct result of my being dyslexic and I suppose in a way a valuable part of it. I've been able to put my aversion to the written word to great effect, operating without language and so breaking down barriers. Those barriers are, of course, in part my own, but there is a sense in which different languages are a barrier to communication for everybody.

Probably because he has managed to overcome his dyslexic problems with relative ease, even to turn them to his own advantage, Charlie is conscious that the affliction can have a positive aspect to it. 'I think the most encouraging thing about being dyslexic is that, in a way, it's like being a left-hander in a right-handed sport,' he said.

> You have an advantage over everybody else because you don't see things the same way as they do. That's why I suppose my work reflects a totally individual technique, style and approach to anima-

tion. There's nothing, in fact, to compare me with. That is I suppose the most encouraging thing for dyslexics, or for people who suffer any kind of disability: they have the opportunity of looking at things from an entirely different perspective from people considered as normal.

Though he was identified at school as having special spelling problems it was not until well into adulthood, when he was involved in making an animated commercial as it happens for the Dyslexia Institute, that Charlie became aware that he was dyslexic. 'To begin with I was horrified,' he recalled.

But quite soon I began to feel encouraged. These problems which I always knew I'd had but had never found an explanation for, never thought much about, suddenly there was a reason for them. It wasn't my fault. I wasn't making anything up. I felt a sense of relief actually.

And, you know, there is an advantage of finding out when you're older. I think that when you're diagnosed at a young age it can be a problem because you might tend to feel you have a problem that you can't overcome. If you're diagnosed as an adult, you might feel slightly bitter because you weren't given proper help and so on, but at least you know that what you've got is something you can overcome. After all, you know you've survived. Mind you, I guess that depends on the degree of dyslexia you have.

Charlie says he knows he will always have problems with dealing with the written word. He has developed a range of strategies to avoid writing things down. His wife does his accounts, his secretary his letters. When dealing with officialdom, for instance in a bank or post office, he is used to running into difficulties. 'I often have to initial a cheque or something like that because I've been going faster than I can just to keep up with other people,' he said. 'The job of coping with being dyslexic is learning not to panic about situations and just living alongside people at your own pace. The biggest problem is not telling people around you to hold on a second because, for instance, it takes you a bit longer to absorb a piece of information.'

IAN MORGAN

Ian Morgan was brought up in a terraced house in Mountain Ash that clings to the side of one of the typically narrow former coal-mining valleys of south Wales. His father was a clerk with the electricity board, his mother a school cook. Education is at a premium in Welsh valley communities and Ian's younger sister did very well at school, passing eight O levels with high grades.

Ian, however, presented problems from the start. He didn't begin at primary school until he was seven because he was asthmatic. And when he did he was placed immediately in the remedial section of the class. 'At Mountain Ash Comprehensive I was told I would never make much of myself because of my spelling,' he recalled. 'When I was fourteen I remember being told I had a reading age of nine.'

He remembers, too, being made fun of a good deal at school and bullied. 'I thought I was just thick,' he said. One of his teachers came to the partial rescue. 'Miss Thomas seemed to sense that I and a couple of other boys regarded as dunces had some ability,' Ian said.

> She encouraged us a lot and put us in for two CSE exams, in History and Religious Education. I passed those and managed to stay on in the sixth form, where I repeated the subjects at O level.
> But it couldn't last. Although I was in the sixth form I was study- ing with the fourth-form class that was doing the subjects. It was obvious that there was no way I was going to make the required sixth-form standard so I left after a year, when I was seventeen.

Soon Ian found a place on a Youth Training Scheme in a large supermarket in nearby Aberdare. There he found himself almost immediately working in the responsible position of storeman, ordering new stock as the old ran out. 'The storeman became ill soon after I arrived,' Ian said. 'I inherited a system and just carried it on, filling in pre-typed sheets with all the headings laid out. But it did me a lot of good. I proved to myself I could do something.'

After six months, however, the training scheme came to an end and he had to leave. Then he found work with Marks & Spencer in Pontypridd, the capital of the valleys, as a relief sales assistant, hired when a full-time person was sick or on holiday. This lasted on and off for four years until he found a temporary job with the Polytechnic of Wales, now the University of Glamorgan, in its printing room. However, this only lasted four months, after which Ian found himself out of work, aged twenty-three, and with ap- parently few prospects.

At this point, realizing he didn't have any qualifications, he decided to have another attempt at full-time education and enrolled at Rhydfelin College of Further Education not far from his home. It was here that one of the lecturers, eyeing his written work, suggested he see Mid Glamorgan County Council's educational psychologist and he discovered he was dyslexic.

'I failed O level English in my first year but re-sat it as a GCSE,' he said.

> I passed because of my course work, not because of the exam. Then I went on to do O level Sociology and Psychology. In my essays I remember getting Bs but passed the exams with a C grade. The same happened when I went on to take them and Religious Education at A level.
>
> I went to see the careers adviser at the college and she suggested I try for university. I said there was no way I could do that because I was dyslexic. She said I might get in as a mature student and suggested I contact Trinity College at Carmarthen.
>
> I remember I tried ringing the college and failed to get through because there was some fault on the line. The operator came on asking what number I wanted. I couldn't remember so I said the university near Carmarthen and so, of course, instead of Trinity College she put me through to St David's University College at Lampeter.
>
> When I asked for a prospectus I was put through to the Department of Theology and Social Studies. I spoke with Marlene, the secretary, and she put me straight through to D. P. Davies, the professor. There I was ringing up a university college out of the blue and straightaway talking to a professor. I couldn't believe it.
>
> I told him what I was looking for and explained that my poor A level grades were because I was dyslexic. By then I had a written reference from my school, saying that if they had recognized I was dyslexic they would have done more for me and I probably would have passed my A levels at that stage.
>
> Anyway, D. P. Davies told me to come down for an interview. I had three interviews in the end, had to read out loud and take dictation, and I was accepted unconditionally. I was twenty-five.

He began studying Social Studies and Environmental Issues, Theology and Welsh Studies, with the first hurdle being to pass the end-of-year exams. 'I found it very hard going at first,' Ian said.

> But my salvation came with the word processor I was able to use in the college. I'd write out my essay in rough, looking up every other word in the dictionary, and then copy it out on the word

processor using its miraculous spellcheck facility. I don't think I would have passed through that first year without the word processor. In my second year my average mark came out at 60 per cent, and then in my final year I met Morffydd, my girlfriend, and she helped me a lot with my grammar.

As part of his degree examination Ian wrote a dissertation on the life of Cardinal Pole, the last Roman Catholic Archbishop of Canterbury, who died within three hours of Mary I in 1559. In his final examinations he was given an extra half an hour and allowed to dictate his answers to an amanuensis, the college chaplain. 'The reason for that was because my handwriting was so awful quite apart from my spelling,' Ian said. 'I was told there might be problems with the external examiner.'

Ian passed his finals with a high-level Lower Second degree, and then took a year off to learn Welsh before becoming a prospective ordinand with the Church in Wales and attending St Michael's Theological College in Cardiff. From being a dunce at school he was looking forward to becoming a vicar in charge of a parish.

'I don't think I'm severely dyslexic because I can read pretty well,' he said.

Mind you, I have to read through a passage twice and study it before I feel confident enough to read in public. So, for instance, the other day I was reading the Bible in church and the word *prisoner* came out as *persons*. My spelling is always going to be awful. You see I still spell phonetically. It's very odd. I can spell words correctly out loud, but when I get to write them down on paper they come out wrong.

The other thing is that I'm naturally left-handed but I write with my right hand, though maybe that was the influence of school making me write 'normally'.

Today, Ian is a confident, humorous man whose character, he readily agrees, has been largely formed by the struggles he has been through as a result of being dyslexic. 'I suppose in a way you could say it was an advantage in the sense that I've come through a kind of suffering and am better able to empathize with people in difficulties,' he said. 'And, of course, that is going to be a big part of my job. At the same time it's difficult not to feel resentful, even a little bitter about it. The other day, for instance, my vicar told me not to dwell on my dyslexia.'

TAKING CHARGE

Cynthia Klein, of Southwark College's Language and Literacy Unit, has observed that students often arrive at the college feeling overwhelmed and at the mercy of their difficulties. Gaining understanding of their problems, she says, is the beginning of having control over them. Although they may need support of one kind or another all their lives, knowing how, where and when to ask for help and precisely what sort of help they need is very different from simply feeling needy and helpless. Two examples of students who have crossed her path make the point.

Pauline was a black Londoner in her early thirties, a single parent and a student at the London College of Fashion. She was referred for a diagnosis and specialist learning support because she was gifted and capable at sewing, pattern cutting and design, yet was unable to pass City and Guilds examinations leading to qualifications.

Pauline could read whatever she needed for the course but was almost completely unable to write because of severe spelling problems. Her tutors were supportive and willing to make up examination-type questions on each week's class work. She would use these as the basis for weekly writing and also make up short sentences or paragraphs using words she felt she particularly needed to learn. 'Pauline learned best by a visual approach,' said Cynthia Klein.

> So, for example, with the word *measure* we linked it with *sure* and then divided it into *me a sure*, using words within words. *Skirt* and *shirt* we linked together, highlighting the *irt* because she did not have much problem with the initial sound.
> *Width* and *length* were more difficult but we divided them as *wid th* and *l eng th*. Though we linked *wide* with *width*, we didn't link *long* with *length* because Pauline got muddled over the vowel change. Waist became *wa is t*, and *button* and *pattern* were learned as *butt on* and *patt ern* because keeping the *tt* together helped her remember the double letters much more easily.

Pauline made up sentences using these words and they were then dictated back to her for practice using sentences such as 'First you measure the length of the skirt' and 'The measurement is from the waist to the hem'. After about six months of weekly work of this kind Pauline passed her first-level examination, gaining confidence

to go on to more advanced levels. 'In Pauline's case it was important to gear the learning programme to her specific needs as that
was where her motivation lay,' said Cynthia Klein.

Rob, another of her students, was from New Zealand and first
attended her learning support class to improve the letters he was
writing home. At the same time he was trying to become a sculptor,
but had failed to get into art college because he didn't have any
O levels. 'I suggested that he began keeping a journal about his art
projects, writing down his ideas and feelings about his work,' said
Cynthia Klein.

> He found writing a slow and arduous task but nevertheless after
> a week brought me the first result, entitled 'The building of the
> spheres'. I could see immediately that in spite of severe spelling and
> writing difficulties there was a great depth of thought and sophistica-
> tion to what he had to say.
>
>   We selected words from the journal for his spelling list, such as
> *sphere, sculpt, sculpture, quality, qualities, properties, experience,
> confidence*, but also *form, build, every*.
>
>   Like Pauline, Rob found a visual approach helpful but because
> he had difficulty in 'tracking' words sequentially; he also found it
> useful to talk about the structure of words, word building and
> prefixes and suffixes and to break up multisyllabic words in this
> way.
>
>   He practised tapping out parts of the word as he said and wrote
> them. In addition I identified awkward and confusing sentences
> which we discussed and he then rewrote them for the following
> week. I also noted and discussed with him *-ed* endings, which he
> tended to omit, and we put this on a checklist for proofreading.
>
>   He continued to keep his art journal which both reinforced spell-
> ings he had learned and generated new words to learn. As new words
> were related to old ones, common letter patterns, word structures
> and endings emerged and were reinforced and reviewed.

Cynthia Klein suggested that Rob think in terms of higher
education and he agreed to take a one-year Fresh Start course at
Southwark College's Adult Education Institute. As a result he was
accepted at art college and eventually graduated with a good second
class degree.

'In Rob's case it was important that all his tutors were able to
identify his potential and to work with him and each other to
ensure that he reached it,' Cynthia Klein said. 'He is also a particularly good example of someone whose initial presentation was of
a person with low-level literacy skills which masked considerable

abilities. These were not revealed until he began writing about his passion, art.'

Cynthia Klein's work illustrates the progress that can be made by adult dyslexics who hitherto have received little or no support. Indeed, as she said, many students often have to 'unlearn' what they have been told before they can advance. Examples she gave were, 'If you read more, your spelling will improve' and 'I can't spell because I don't pronounce words right'. 'One student told me she had enjoyed using long words at school until a teacher told her not to use long words until she could spell the short ones,' Cynthia Klein recalled. 'That was the end of her writing career.'

It is plain, therefore, that effective help can be given to dyslexic adults, so long as it is intelligently focused and, most importantly, geared individually to their specific needs and problems. As ever, it is a question of persuading those in need that it is possible for them, with adequate support and encouragement, to help themselves. They *can* take charge of a condition that previously was controlling them and determining their life's destiny.

Chapter 4

Families

There is general agreement amongst those who have researched and studied dyslexia that, because it is genetically determined, it runs in families. For instance, Dr Beve Hornsby, who was in charge of the Dyslexia Clinic at St Bartholomew's Hospital in London during the 1970s, reported that 88 per cent of the children seen there had a family history of dyslexia. The chance that a child of a dyslexic parent will also be dyslexic is reckoned to be about one in four.

It is also generally accepted by specialists that a dyslexic person's brain cells are arranged differently to a greater or lesser degree from those of other people. 'Since you inherit your brain cell arrangement in much the same way as you inherit aspects of your personality and your physical characteristics, it is not surprising that so many dyslexics have close family with the condition,' says Dr Hornsby.

The fact that dyslexia is inherited and so runs in families has a number of practical implications that hitherto have been little considered. First of all is the potential for guilt amongst parents who, however involuntarily, pass on dyslexia to their children. The fact that there is no deliberate intention involved is neither here nor there if that is, in fact, what some parents feel.

Secondly, there is the strong likelihood that dyslexic people will grow up in families where more than one person is dyslexic. This can have advantages and disadvantages. When these are pointed out they can seem obvious. For instance, there is a greater chance of sympathetic understanding between siblings and parents and children where first-hand experience of dyslexia is shared. On the other hand, all the problems associated with dyslexia, such as frustration and disorganization, can all too easily be compounded and made worse whenever two or more dyslexics are gathered together. They can be doubly compounded where, for whatever reason, dyslexia is denied.

The following profiles of families where more than one member is dyslexic provides ample evidence of these and other factors. The more such dimensions of dyslexia are understood and catered for the easier the lives of dyslexic people will become.

THE SPENCERS

Yvonne Spencer, the only member of her family who is not dyslexic, recounted the following incident with her eldest son when asked to explain what it is like living with dyslexia inside a family:

> Ben just threw a wobbly about one of his essays. He had spent three-quarters of an hour poring over this question trying to understand it. Then he spent three hours doing it. But when he came to read back what he had done he found he couldn't understand his answer.
>
> The final straw came when he discovered he had answered question 2 instead of question 5 because he couldn't read his own notes. So he had a blow-out, stomping around, screaming and shouting. This kind of thing we take in our stride, I suppose. The only good thing is that the family knows what is going on and so doesn't over-react.

After attending a series of special schools, Ben was studying Computer Science at home to add to his A levels in Maths and Economics. His sister Sophie, seven years younger, was spending the week at a special school but returning home at weekends. Yvonne's husband, Gordon, a graphic designer, discovered only late in life that he was dyslexic. However, looking back he now sees dyslexia as the explanation for countless problems and incidents.

Since Ben was a small child Yvonne and Gordon Spencer have faced a series of battles with their local education authority to have their children recognized as dyslexic, Statemented and provided with special help. They have had to resort to taking in student lodgers, help from charitable foundations and even using an insurance settlement for water flooding in their house to pay school fees. Yvonne makes the point that living with severely dyslexic children is quite a different matter from coping with children who are mildly or moderately affected and who, with adequate support, can usually manage within the state education system. 'With many dyslexic children I suppose you can get through with a lot of extra help,' she said.

> But with a severely dyslexic child, it would be like sending a blind child to a normal school and throwing away the braille books. Inevitably you would end up with behavioural and emotional problems. The stress is enormous. You really have no choice, absolutely no choice whatsoever, but to send a child like that to a specialist school.
>
> Of course, it's a wrench to send them away from home, and if you haven't got the money and you have to struggle with the local authority to provide help, it's a financial nightmare. On top of that if your partner is severely dyslexic as well, then obviously you're lacking support in dealing with the authorities, filling in the forms, writing the endless letters. It is difficult. It can be very, very hard.

Yvonne and Gordon met at a party in London. 'I went with some friends,' Yvonne recalled.

> He was playing the guitar gently in the background which quite impressed me. Then he produced this business card and so I thought, he's reasonably OK and we started going out together.
>
> Gordon was incredibly vague, but then I'd never been out with an artistic person before. I'd always gone out with estate agents, stockbrokers and accountants, and so I rather thought it was the arty side of him when he turned up on the wrong day, at the wrong time, and in the wrong place – several times running, actually. But it really was rather confusing, to begin with at any rate. I mean, you remind someone at 4 o'clock in the afternoon that you're meeting outside Harrods in London at 8.30 pm. Then that evening you're standing there for about two hours in the freezing cold, in February, and it's snowing. Meanwhile, Gordon has actually gone to Peter Jones, waited for five minutes and returned home, because he knows he probably got it wrong.
>
> One thing I never really could cope with was when I telephoned him from the office with a message. Looking back I know that he was impatient, because he obviously needed to write it down to remember, and write it down slowly. But, of course, I was in a hurry, I was running my own estate management business. So,

anyway, I would just phone up, say something quickly, and inevitably the message would be totally lost. Phone messages are still a problem.

Yvonne and Gordon nearly didn't get married because of this hidden dyslexia. After they had become engaged Yvonne went abroad with a girlfriend on a prearranged holiday. During the fortnight away she wrote to Gordon, but didn't receive a reply until the last day.

> The only reason I got the letter was the fact that the coach was two hours late taking us to to the airport. When I picked it up I took one look and thought this engagement is off when I get home, this is no love letter.
>
> I mean, it was half a page of very basic scrawl. Looking at it now, and I've kept it – it's the only letter I've ever had from Gordon – the language is extraordinarily simple for an intelligent person, with sentences like, 'I went to work today. I worked hard.' Now I know what dyslexia is I can see why he did that. Writing such a basic message with such simple words meant there wouldn't be spelling mistakes. Gordon told me later that it took him an enormously long time to write that letter.

'It's a strange thing,' said Gordon, 'I can draw, but I can't write. I had a very basic secondary modern education which in its own way was fine for me because it wasn't too demanding. What changed my life was going to art school. I think there were a lot of dyslexic people there actually, so I was in good company. Half of them couldn't spell either.'

Early on Yvonne and Gordon slipped into a routine in which she did all the household paperwork, dealing with bills, filling in forms. 'It's not just a problem with the writing and spelling,' Yvonne said. 'It's a result of a lack of organizational skills as well.'

Dyslexia as a word entered their lives when their first child, Ben, was seven. Because he was an asthmatic and a hyperactive child he was already in a small private school in Richmond and in a class two years behind his peer group. But it was increasingly plain that there were more fundamental problems. Ben was assessed at the Victoria Developmental Centre, which specializes in hyperactive, slow-learning children. Yvonne and Gordon raised a second mortgage on their home to have him taught at the Victoria Centre.

After a year he had settled down and seemed to be making progress so they moved him back into primary school in Richmond.

'It was an excellent school, with sympathetic teachers, but Ben just fell apart,' said Yvonne. 'He had to be be dragged to school, kicking and screaming.'

There ensued a long-drawn-out and exhausting struggle to persuade the local education authority to make a Statement identifying Ben's special needs. Meanwhile he was sent to a succession of private specialist boarding schools. Eventually after four years the LEA relented, made a Statement and began contributing towards the costs of Ben's special education. However, each year remained a knife-edge problem so far as funding was concerned. The money from the LEA was never enough, and the Spencers had to bridge the gap with their own money and also raise money from charities. 'At one point I wrote around to a hundred foundations,' said Yvonne.

Meanwhile she attended a dyslexia course at the Richmond Dyslexia Association and quickly realized that here was also the explanation for Gordon's problems. Then came Sophie. Immediately she began at primary school there was a familiar pattern of stress, frustration, panic and temper tantrums. 'When Sophie was diagnosed at six years old I knew we had ten years to go,' said Yvonne.

Because of her elder brother I knew exactly what the problems would be. She had this very white terrified little face going off in the morning and then when we reached the school gates, she would start singing and being very bright and smiling. But it was all a façade. At the end of the day I'd pick her up and this little monster would appear. After tears and tantrums she'd have exhausted herself and be settled down in front of the television. She'd have supper and then go off to bed where she'd actually go to sleep for a while.

But then, come 10 or 11 o'clock, or even midnight, I'd go into her room and there she'd be trying to teach herself to read, sitting on the floor staring at her books. I'd sit with her, with a large gin and tonic, and listen, just listen to it all pour out. She'd say to me, 'It's better no one knows, Mummy, it just causes me more trouble.'

It was absolutely heartbreaking. I felt I was committing child abuse sending her to school. Eventually she'd go off to sleep again, but often wake up in the middle of the night with nightmares. Sometimes she'd wet the bed. And in the morning the whole process would begin again – the white face, 'I've got a headache mummy', 'I don't feel well mummy', 'I've got tummy aches again mummy' . . .

There followed six years when the Spencers attempted unsuccessfully to persuade their local education authority to make a Statement about Sophie's special needs and, like Ben, send her to a special school. However, despite a successful appeal to the Secretary of State for Education to have the matter reconsidered no progress was made.

'The situation is crazy,' said Yvonne.

> There is an Act of Parliament which states the legal position of the child but throughout the country the various local authorities interpret it exactly as they like. One child at Sophie's school living literally across the river from us is Statemented and paid for. Another child was Statemented in just six months by the Bournemouth authorities. Had we known we would have moved there.
>
> At the end of the day it's the money. The longer they delay the less they have to pay. Often it seems they are willing to Statement mildly dyslexic children because they know they can cope with them inside the mainstream school system. But severely dyslexic children have to be sent away, with all the attendant costs.

The Spencers did send Sophie to a specialist school, but at enormous personal financial sacrifice, never knowing from one term to the next where the money was going to come from. Charities made all the difference, together with borrowing money from friends and with schools providing bursaries or waiving fees at critical moments. Even so it was a wearing process, time-consuming, often humiliating, and a continual strain. 'Statementing is important to us not just because of the money,' said Yvonne.

> But so that we can feel Sophie is protected if anything goes wrong. What would happen, for instance, if I was to fall under a bus or Gordon had a heart attack? As it is it looks as though Sophie will have been through most stages of her school life before all the legal processes are worked through and the local authority is forced to make a Statement of her special needs. I've been warned that it could well take until she is fifteen. Meanwhile we somehow have to find the £15,000 a year it takes to keep her at her weekly boarding school.

Gordon Spencer has had his own problems coming to terms not just with his children's problems but with the fact that he himself is dyslexic. He admitted that he delayed having himself properly assessed for many years because he was afraid of what the results might show. 'They might have concluded that I wasn't dyslexic at all and confirmed my own feelings that I was simply inadequate so far as writing is concerned,' he said. As it was he was assessed as being dyslexic with an IQ of 129.

Gordon said he had difficulty, especially during the early years, in relating to the children's problems, partly because he was often working late, but partly because he didn't appreciate that he himself was dyslexic. 'I think I would have been more sympathetic if I had,' he said.

> Still, I remember one incident with Ben which made me realize how he felt. I was asked to go with him on a school trip to one of the London museums because of his asthma. In the museum the kids were given a list of questions and I followed Ben and a friend around looking at the exhibits, reading what was said and answering questions. I remember seeing Ben's face and realized that he was panicking – absolutely panicking – because, of course, he hadn't a clue. He couldn't read the questions, couldn't read about the exhibits, and of course his partner was getting cross with him. You could see he was absolutely terrified.
>
> I think that's probably how Sophie felt most of the time, too – sheer fear.

Reflecting on the strains within dyslexic families, Yvonne spoke in turn about her husband and children. An added problem for them was unemployment, with Gordon being made redundant.

> My husband's confidence was zapped years ago and it's only now, aged fifty, that he is beginning to come to terms with it and get help. For him it's like opening the door of an Aladdin's cave. Everyone else was in there and he was outside. Now there is a possibility for him to go through the door as well and he is excited and positively obsessive about it.
>
> It's going to be a long, hard and slow business for him, learning to spell even quite simple words and do things without relying on me. He is on a computer course, braving a jobs club, and trying for a retraining course. It all sounds pretty ordinary for an unemployed person these days, but for him it's like trying to climb Everest without the proper equipment. There's that strong element of fear with him all the time, fear of ridicule and fear of falling, falling and never getting up again.
>
> That might sound melodramatic but every adult dyslexic I know has said the same thing. Then there's the added problem of knowing your child's dyslexia comes from you and you can't do anything about it, let alone knowing you don't have enough money to help your child. It's as if there were a series of eye operations which could

help your child see normally, but the health authorities hadn't the resources and you couldn't raise the money either.

The stress inevitably extends to the children, however hard you attempt to shield them from it. I can see that Ben's studies are being affected. Having been messed about by the system himself he certainly doesn't want his sister to suffer and he is too old not to understand what a dreadful struggle we had helping him.

He feels guilty, even about needing money for a pair of jeans. He told me once that he is never going to have children himself. He doesn't want them to suffer. Actually, as I keep telling him, he's a great success. He passed good enough A levels to get into university. More importantly, he is a stable, caring and useful member of society. Although it's going to be a struggle all the way for him, he's lucky in comparison with his father, who was never diagnosed as a child. He's confident enough now when dealing with forms to write 'Sorry it's a mess, I'm dyslexic', or when answering the phone to ask people to repeat a message.

With Sophie the problem is the heartbreak of wanting her to be at home but knowing she needs special education and having no money to provide it. Every family facing the problem of unemployment knows what it is like to worry about money and the future, wondering where the next term's school fees will come from. Living from month to month inevitably takes its toll.

And Sophie is very perceptive about things, which can make it worse. There was an advert on television the other day, for a magazine which had a special feature on stress. 'You should buy that,' Sophie told me. And I thought I was putting on a good act! Mind you, Sophie knows little of the fight we've had to make on her behalf. She thinks my stress is related to unemployment.

The legal battle to get Sophie what is rightfully hers has taken on farcical proportions, with the authorities arguing about what she was like seven years ago. For us during these seven years it has been as though our lives have been put on hold. And the question is still not resolved.

Some days I cry behind closed doors, away from family and friends. Other days I get angry and walk furiously around the park until I'm too tired to storm into the council offices and create a scene. Then when something happens like seeing Sophie happy in her school, taking a part in the school play, or hearing a friend say how much she has improved, I pick myself up and fight on, determined that if we end up living in a tent, Sophie will have the chance that every normal child has.

But often in this situation you feel as though you're living continuously with fear: Will we cope? Will I crack up? Will our marriage survive? I know from the people I have met over the years that the divorce rate is very high in marriages where one partner is dyslexic.

I think it's easier on the family if it's the mother rather than the father who is dyslexic. You tend to depend so much more on the husband as the wage earner for a start and the pressures there can be enormously high, with problems at work as well as at home. A wife and mother who is dyslexic may have her own problems, the house may be a bit chaotic, but often it's very homely. Often, too, the husbands of dyslexic women seem to be high-powered, very good at sorting things out.

If the dyslexic partner in a marriage can be based at home, life is generally much easier. Since Gordon has been unemployed he has more time to play with Sophie. While I take the load of the legal battle, he has had more time to be relaxed with her.

And it's not all a tragic story by any means. Life is never dull with dyslexic people. We have some hilarious stories to tell. I'm very proud of my family. We've stuck together through thick and thin.

THE SPIERSES

Families who live with dyslexia are always on the lookout for breakthroughs. One came for the Spiers family, who live in Melksham in Wiltshire, when Mark caught his first bus to Bath. He was fourteen years old.

'I was amazed,' said his mother Jackie, who is also dyslexic.

He came home with a timetable, worked out the different numbers and the different-colour buses, and said, 'I'm off.' Then, just as he was going out of the door I remembered, and said, 'You will cross by the road by the bank?' He looked puzzled and answered, 'Why do I want to cross the road?' I replied, 'You have to go on the other side of the road because the bus that you want will be going the other way.' He thought for a moment then nodded. I had visions of him waiting interminably on the wrong side of the road.

I was frantic with worry. How would he find his way round the bus station in Bath? It's a pretty big one, you know. Well in the end he got home OK and I asked him how he'd managed. 'Mum, I asked at the information desk,' he said. I was so proud of him.

Mark has a brother, Noel, who is two years older, and a sister, Anna, three years younger. Like their mother, all are severely dyslexic. Yet it was many years before Jackie or her husband, William, discovered the full extent of the problem. Jackie, in fact, was a classic example of a hidden dyslexic, the condition hidden even from herself. By the time she and William, a haulage contractor, met she had evolved a whole series of strategies to avoid being faced with a panic attack whenever forced to read a menu, write a cheque or even offer directions. 'I was lucky,' she said:

> I went to a private convent school in Bath and somehow slipped through the lessons without too much difficulty. Of course, I had all the usual problems with trying to read aloud in class. I just wouldn't do it. Eventually one of them did get me to read after a fashion, by painstakingly going over things. Five minutes into an English lesson I'd ask to go to the bathroom. I'd go out and be twenty minutes. Of course, I was only messing around outside. It worked every time.
>
> I liked tennis and PE, needlework and cooking. Otherwise I just messed around and enjoyed the social side. I always had a friend with me, especially going to school and coming home. My one big fear was missing the bus because I wasn't sure which one to catch. I remember panicking if the bus went on a detour because, of course, I didn't know where it was going.
>
> I used to stay in a lot at home because to go anywhere from our house you had to catch a bus and I couldn't because I didn't know which one. So I never went anywhere. Looking back, my mum helped a lot. I've always had someone to lean on – first my mum and now William.

Instead of insisting she attempt any exams in school her parents managed to find a place for her on a Catering and Community Care Course at Trowbridge Further Education College. 'I stayed there as long as I possibly could,' Jackie said. 'I never passed an exam but just muffled along from one course to the next. I did quite well in practical catering, which boosted my confidence.'

When she was twenty she met William and they were married within a year. 'William didn't realize that I was different in any way,' Jackie said. 'I thought, this guy can look after me.' 'Obviously we were very attracted to each other,' said William. 'At first I was unaware of any problems, but gradually they unfolded, though it was a long way into our marriage. I didn't twig that it was necessary for me to do all the accounts, the cheques and all the other bits and pieces that I suppose other couples get involved with together.'

'William liked being in charge of everything so I just let him carry on,' said Jackie. 'He gave me cash every week. Every so often he would say, "Don't you think you ought to have a cheque book?" and I'd say, "No, no, just give me the money." That's how it went on for ages. William even did the Christmas cards.'

'Every Christmas Jackie would say that my handwriting was far neater and so would I mind doing them,' said William.

> Of course, I didn't work out that Jackie was absolutely overfaced at writing the Christmas cards, doing the lists and getting the addresses. In those days, too, I was working very long hours and, partly because of that I think, our marriage went very well in the early years. We had lots of friends, went out a lot.

The problems started when their first child, Noel, and later Mark started school. 'I remember William was very relaxed about it at first,' Jackie said.

> He felt sure they would catch up. But I suppose I related it to my own experience at school. Suddenly I couldn't cope with reliving with my own children what I'd been through as a child. Somehow it was worse than living through it myself. The teachers would say, 'Oh, he'll be all right.' But I'd seen it all before. As a child you float through. You don't know the implications.

Noel, the eldest child, managed with special help within the state system, taking GCSEs two years late. However, managing in this way with Mark proved impossible. 'Noel began to read when he was eight, and I hadn't until I was twelve, so I suppose I felt that was an advance,' said Jackie.

> But Mark was worse. At five I was the only one who could understand him talking. He'd cry a lot at school. He used to break pencils and scribble in books, out of sheer frustration. He knew he could do things in theory but when it came to putting things down on paper he just couldn't. He would sit there at his desk staring at a piece of paper, somehow bottling it all up inside himself. That went on for four years until the teachers began to get concerned.

Mark was assessed and found to be dyslexic. There followed a long battle with the local education authority to have him Statemented and sent away to a special school.

To begin with Mark had special one-to-one help at school for five hours a week. But this did not work well. He became upset at being taken out of the classroom. 'He finds any change of routine difficult, even now,' said Jackie.

The Spierses appealed against the LEA's decision not to make a Statement, taking the case on appeal to the Secretary of State for Education. Eventually, after a battle lasting more than two years, they won their case and the LEA agreed to pay Mark's fees at a private specialist school.

'The problem was lack of resources,' said William.

They were very conscious of setting a precedent. If they did it for one child would it have to be done for others with specific learning difficulties? And I think they regarded us as middle-class pushy parents, probably making too much fuss over a problem that would come right of its own accord if only we persevered.

The arguments with the local authority and the appeal were a nerve-racking and upsetting process. It took a lot of heartache, a lot of time, and needless to say a lot of money.

Mark became a changed child as a result of going away to school during the week. 'We miss him, of course, and he doesn't enjoy being away from home. But he realizes it's the best thing for him because he's so much calmer,' said Jackie.

I always remember his coming home one weekend after about six weeks and one of those little things happened that used to trigger him off into one of his rages. He stood there in the middle of the kitchen and I thought, 'Oh God, here we go.' Then he stopped, and I said, 'Are you all right now?' and he answered, 'It's all right, mummy. They've taught me to control my temper tantrums. They get me to relax.'

Another blow hit the family, however, when Anna was discovered to be dyslexic as well. 'It was the end because I really thought she was going to be fine,' said Jackie.

I just couldn't believe it. That for me was the worst moment. I thought, being a female, she would be all right. Perhaps she might have been like Noel and more or less coped, but to discover she was worse even than Mark was a bombshell.

I put a block on it, in fact, whereas by then William knew we were going to have to go through it all again. There she was, seven years old, in a state at school, still not reading, not even knowing the days of the week. It was classic.

It was at this point that Jackie began to admit to herself that she too was dyslexic. A turning point came when she attempted to help Anna with some simple maths homework. 'I did the first two questions and was quite pleased with myself,' she said. 'Then Anna's friend came for tea and finished them off. When the work came back from school it was with the first two answers completely wrong and all the rest marked excellent. I just burst into tears.'

William and Jackie Spiers had another three-year battle with the local education authority, which went to another appeal to the Secretary of State for Education and then a threat of judicial review, before Anna was placed in a special school. Today the family are approaching some kind of normality where dyslexia is not completely ruling their lives.

Jackie is attending literacy classes and finally learning to read properly. She has also found aerobics helpful. 'It gives me confidence,' she said. 'It somehow synchronizes my co-ordination. When I first started I was all over the place. Now if I miss a few classes I start feeling insecure again.'

William has become chairman of the Mid-Wiltshire Dyslexia Association, edits its newsletter, runs a telephone helpline and is also on the executive committee of the British Dyslexia Association. 'There was a period when the whole of our family life revolved around the problems of dyslexia,' he recalled.

> In the early years when we knew very little about it we were often at a loss about what to do. Sometimes, when the children were younger and we were going through the mill with the education authorities trying to get help we would become totally frustrated.
>
> Now, some years on, we're getting things more into perspective. You learn to get a balance into life. And, you know, dyslexia is not all bad. The ways the children and Jackie think just amazes me sometimes. They'll put a totally different perspective on a subject that completely throws me, which is good because it makes me see life in a different way.'

'I would like to have a lot more self-confidence,' said Jackie.

> I would love to be able to just sit down and write a letter to a friend without having to worry about the punctuation, the spelling and the writing. Trying to concentrate on all three at once means I end up just not doing it. So I've taught myself to type on a computer, which has opened a big door. Now I've got to get myself a bit more relaxed about spelling, not worry quite so much, and use the dictionary more. Mind you I find using a dictionary difficult. It takes me so long to find the word I'm searching for that I often look up the wrong beginnings. As long as the letters at the beginning are all right you're OK, but if you're looking up the wrong beginnings you can spend forever looking up the word and never finding it.
>
> I'd love to be able to help William with his business a bit more. Whether he'd actually allow me to I don't know. But it would be nice to do something that is for myself. When that day will be I don't know. Slowly, slowly we'll see.

THE HOLLIDAYS

'I hated school myself,' said Gill Holliday. 'I went to a girls' high school, and had this particularly horrid teacher. On my sixteenth birthday I went into school, took my things out of my desk, stood up and said, "Right, I'm off!" I remember the teacher chasing me down the corridor and shouting, "Stop! You can't go, it's against the law!" '

Gill Holliday is used to taking things into her own hands. Characteristically, she refused to be browbeaten as her two small sons in turn faced difficulty at school. When she tried to persuade teachers and her local education authority that there was a problem which needed special attention she was faced with a blank wall of indifference and hostility. So she took her children out of school and started educating them at home.

The Holliday family is, by self-identification, working class. More than that, it is supremely confident, has little time for authority, is sceptical about the advantages of academic attainment, and is convinced that there are many alternative routes to happiness. In all these respects it is far from typical. None the less, the family's experience of dyslexia is instructive.

They live on a small, five-acre holding on the edge of Carlton village near Barnsley in Yorkshire. Geoff Holliday is a lorry driver, and as with many such families leaves most of the decisions regarding the upbringing of his two young sons, Geoffrey and Andrew, to his wife Gill.

She remembers that when Geoffrey first went to nursery school he enjoyed it. 'There were no literacy skills involved at that stage and it was great,' she said.

> But as soon as he moved into the reception class of the infant school the problems started and steadily got worse over three years.
>
> The teacher claimed he was learning to read, but he was memorizing the books he had. The teachers kept saying he would eventually be all right. Then they said he was lazy. He was kept in at playtimes and he used to just sit there, watching everybody else through the window. He became a withdrawn, frightened, timid child at school. But once he was at home he was completely different. He'd be full of confidence and happy once he was outside, playing with his motorbike.
>
> I became really angry and frustrated at not being able to put my finger on what was obviously a problem. There seemed no

explanation for it. I felt as though we'd lost the battle before it had even started. I just felt powerless as a mother. It was an awful thing, having to send your child to school and knowing that once he was there he would have a dreadful time.

In desperation I went to see the headteacher and she gave me the number of a private tutor. But she never once said that Geoffrey could be assessed by the local education authority and receive extra help at school. I think her attitude was that it was our fault as parents, because we weren't bookish at home. She didn't really believe Geoffrey had a problem.

The meeting with the headteacher provided the breakthrough, however, since the private tutor she recommended had been trained at the Dyslexia Institute at the University College of North Wales, Bangor. She assessed Geoffrey and pronounced that 'This child is amongst the worst cases of dyslexia I've seen, but his anxiety is far worse than his dyslexia.' The Hollidays began to pay for him to have private lessons, twice a week.

Meanwhile, Geoffrey's brother Andrew was starting school and undergoing a similar educational experience. When Gill saw him losing confidence and the school once again refusing to accept that there was a problem she decided to act. She took both children out of school and started teaching them at home.

'I decided that the school had been a failure, not the children,' she said.

I felt that if they stayed in school they'd come out feeling they were failures and that's no way to begin your life. I decided that since the system couldn't adjust to them there was no way they were going to be labelled failures when plainly they are not. They are both bright boys and taught in the right way they will be able to make good progress in the essential basic skills. I think my best option is to encourage them in the things they do best and adapt the method of teaching in a more practical direction rather than putting continual pressure and emphasis on paper work.

Geoffrey and Andrew go for an hour twice a week to the private tutor, who sets them work to be done at home. Gill teaches them for an hour and a half each morning, mainly Maths and English, and the rest of the day is their own, working and playing on the smallholding. 'It took three years for Geoffrey to regain his self-confidence,' Gill said. 'He was so used to trying and failing at school that he had just given up. I am confident I have done the right thing and the method of teaching is working. The tutor is impressed at how much both boys have progressed since being taken out of school.'

The private lessons cost the Holliday family £40 a week, an amount they afford mainly as a result of not having a mortgage on their mobile home. The family have been involved in a long-running battle with the local education authority to persuade it to provide appropriate special help for the children and, when that was not forthcoming, to persuade it that the children were being properly taught at home.

The LEA found a fierce and formidable opponent in Gill Holliday. Around her coalesced more than seventy families in South Yorkshire with similar problems. Many meetings have been held, petitions raised, MPs involved, delegations sent to the House of Commons, and on-going press and television interest attracted. The result has been a gradual modification in the LEA's attitude, with piecemeal extra provision made for children with special needs.

Meanwhile the Holliday children have been getting on with their lives. Gill Holliday is confident that they will find practical work, such as farming or following in the family tradition of scrap metal merchants. 'Sometimes I worry that we're not pushing them towards an academic career,' she said. 'Sometimes I think we should be more like other parents and be anxious for our children to go to college. But really I don't mind what they do so long as they try their best and they're happy.'

THE GREENS

Louise Green, asked to describe what it is like to live in a dyslexic family, told the following story. She and her three children, John (then aged thirteen), Sarah (eleven) and Ben (seven) - all of them, like herself, dyslexic - were making their way through a crush of people on London's Underground.

Coming out of a pedestrian tunnel the path divided with one sign pointing to the Central Line and another indicating the Circle Line. 'I remember saying to the children, "Come on, we've got to make for the Circle Line." Of course, we misread the signs and unhesitatingly we all went down the passage heading for the Central Line.'

Their 'dyslexic day' did not end there. They were travelling to keep an appointment with a specialist doctor in central London. When they finally arrived in Harley Street Louise fumbled in her handbag and realized with a shock that she had left her notebook at home. This is a vital piece of her equipment. In it she records detailed names and numbers which otherwise she invariably forgets. So, here they were, near their destination but unable to recall the name of the doctor they were supposed to see or the number of the building where he practised.

'I remembered that the doctor had an odd name beginning with "Fore . . .",' Louise said. 'So we were reduced to wandering up and down the road looking at the nameplates on the doors to see if there was a name bearing any resemblance to that. Finally, we asked at a group practice. The receptionist looked in a doctors' handbook and found a Dr Forecast practising two doors away.'

Coping with such an exasperating series of events is particularly galling for the Green family since they are, in fact, exceptionally intelligent. Louise herself, whose personal story is related in Chapter 1, has a very high IQ rating of 158 (average 100). John has an IQ of 142 and the other children are well above average as well. 'We suffer from being to the severe side of average dyslexia, counterbalanced by our high intelligence,' said Louise.

Exceptionally high intelligence has its obvious advantages. However, where the children are concerned it means that they have not qualified for any special help in school since their reading age has always more or less corresponded to their chronological age.

John, the eldest child, was discovered to be dyslexic when he was eight. 'He was having enormous problems,' Louise said.

> Somehow he couldn't retain visual patterns in his mind. The teacher told me he was educationally subnormal, though as we later discovered he had a reasoning age three years above his chronological age.
>
> From six and a half years old he was unhappy at school and had temper tantrums at home. He would go rigid and refuse to go to school. He complained of stomach aches all the time, though there was nothing wrong as far as our doctor could tell. I didn't realize that stress in children can make them physically ill.

Eventually the family's general practitioner recommended they took John to see an educational psychologist, who diagnosed him as dyslexic. Louise, a teacher, then attended a course at the South

Watford Dyslexia Unit and as a result soon realized that she was dyslexic herself, as were her other children. 'First of all my heart plummeted,' she recalled.

But then I felt as though someone had lifted a weight from my shoulders. Up to then I had always felt that I was simply stupid.

I was delighted, too, that we had found an explanation for John's behaviour. The educational psychologist explained that his temper tantrums were triggered by extreme frustration caused by the discrepancy between what he wanted to do and what he was actually capable of doing. It meant that he didn't have any major psychiatric problems. Now we knew what the problem was we could organize the help to put it right.

Looking back I can now see why he was becoming frustrated, for instance when he tried and failed to do things he saw me doing, like stack bricks in a pile. He was a terribly messy eater. We would have to spread a groundsheet under his high chair and bath him straight afterwards – another sign of his poor co-ordination.

Although he spoke fluently from eighteen months, so we actually had conversations, he couldn't follow lists of instructions. And he hated getting dressed in the morning and undressed at night. He would run around the upstairs of the house screaming and crying. He found tying his shoelaces so difficult that I threaded elastic through the lace-holes so he could slip his shoes on and off.

Though it was a relief to discover John was dyslexic I wasn't so pleased when we worked out that our middle child was dyslexic as well. By then we knew how badly the state education system failed bright dyslexics and that she would get little help for her problems.

I knew that our third child was dyslexic before he even started school. But his teacher was very understanding and helpful, so it wasn't until he was in his fourth year that his problems really began.

The two boys are very easily discouraged. When they were at primary school they were prepared to send in messy, scrappy and almost illegible work. They didn't like to concentrate for long periods and it was very difficult to get them to settle down to homework. Often they spent twice as long trying to avoid doing their work as the work actually takes, using tactics from temper tantrums to shutting themselves in their bedrooms.

Sarah is totally different. She is far more motivated and will spend hours on her homework, constantly wanting it checked and rechecked, and writing it out several times. In fact she is too much of a perfectionist and would make life easier for herself if she didn't worry so much. She says that she finds it irritating and frustrating when she can't remember how to spell certain words, even ones that she has already written earlier on the page.

Except for the very occasional flare-up Sarah is coping well and at least appears self-contained and content. Of course, appearances can mislead and while a child seems well-balanced, parents are reluctant to rock the boat. Girls often fall through the net in this way. Because they conform and *seem* to be coping no one notices or makes a fuss. When they eventually erupt – usually in their teens – this is often put down to 'hormones' and development problems.

Louise's husband, Malcolm, who is away from home a good deal with his job, advising on garage design, says he was often completely baffled by much of his wife's behaviour in the early days of their marriage. He remembers that Louise became a different person when, at the age of thirty-three, she discovered she was dyslexic. 'Until then she was forever apologizing for things, always assuming she was in the wrong,' he said. 'Suddenly she acquired a lot more confidence.'

Louise said that she thought it was less strain on a marriage if the partner who was dyslexic was the one who remained at home.

> The strain on the main wage earner to perform well at all times or else fear the loss of their job would be tremendous, as would be forever covering up for apparent inadequacies. It is also better for the dyslexic parent to be at home to deal with the children, with whom they can share experiences. Forgetfulness at home can be embarrassing, of course, but it tends not to be disastrous or expensive.

Out of school the problems of dealing with the two boys and with Sarah have proved different. 'With Sarah it has mostly been her unhappiness caused by feelings of self-worthlessness and what she terms her *stupidity*,' said Louise.

> But the boys have been hardest to deal with. Although I sympathize with the frustration behind temper tantrums and screaming fits, no family can survive if they let these rule the roost.
>
> At primary school the two boys were definitely out of kilter with their peer group and got on better with friends out of their own age range, either older or younger. Periodically this led to problems at school, though not so much at home where it was easier for them to choose their friends.
>
> When John, the eldest, was at his lowest ebb the other two were too little to interfere. They could be settled with a video or put to bed, while we coped with the eldest one. Now Ben has reached this stage and it is made much worse by John interfering, telling us what we should do with him, that we aren't being fair because we treated *him* differently, and generally winding up his little brother.
>
> I think it's true to say that John has had the hardest time of all. Because he was the first it was years before we spotted there was

a problem. We spent a couple of years trying to identify it and another three years learning how to put it right. It's amazing to me that he has come through that experience and is as nice as he is today. Seven years on from when we discovered his dyslexia he is almost a model pupil and in no way resembles the monster he used to be. He still gets twitchy over any changes to his routine, but generally he is improving all the time.

Still, life can be intensely frustrating for the children and as I don't always say what I mean we can all end up getting totally confused. It can be difficult because the boys and I are extremely disorganized. They can't rely on me to remind them of the things they need for school and I can't rely on them to tell me when there are notes from school or when they need to take extra things like sports gear.

When they do remember to tell me they typically choose the worst possible time, like when I'm cooking or on the phone. So I forget completely and later they chorus very self-righteously that they had told me. Then I feel cross or guilty depending on my mood and either try to blame them or feel useless.

Our disorganization means that we are always losing things we need urgently, like car keys or homework. For, of course, we never remember which 'safe place' we have used. It is also difficult because, like many disabilities, dyslexia is always worse when the person is tired or under pressure. A family unit tends to experience tiredness and pressure together, which compounds the problem.

Another major difficulty is that verbal or phone messages either don't get passed on at all, or else get passed on inaccurately. I can be as guilty as the children if I don't write a message down. Verbal messages somehow become confused and what one person says, even if accurate, isn't always what another hears. Failing to remember what one has said to one person and then saying something different to another is a constant occurrence. On the other hand there is a lot of laughter because when things go wrong there is usually a funny side. Dyslexics are frequently quite original and life is rarely dull.

Because the dyslexic child finds reading and writing difficult they tend to get used to concentrating harder and can frequently become outstanding in their chosen field. I think it's beneficial having more than one dyslexic person in a family because then the sufferer doesn't feel the odd one out and is less likely to feel alienated. Having a dyslexic parent in the family is helpful, too, because they can better understand why their children do what they do and either sympathize or offer practical help such as learning strategies. They are also best placed to stop a child getting away with the phrase, 'I can't do that because I'm dyslexic . . .'.

In our family being dyslexic has had some benefits. The children have learnt to be self-reliant from an earlier age than usual, out of sheer necessity. They are not over-protected and they have learnt one vital lesson early on – that life isn't fair. They have developed their own specialist skills. They have learnt not to judge by appearances. And I think they are more aware of other people's feelings because they are so conscious of their own.

Although I know it is not my fault that the children are dyslexic, sometimes I do feel guilty because I know they have inherited it from me. I feel guilty as well because I know what a struggle they will have with some aspects of their school work. I get very frustrated that the special help children need isn't available in the state sector unless their work falls significantly below their chronological age.

THE FAMILY DYNAMICS OF DYSLEXIA

As Tolstoy memorably remarked, at the opening of his novel *Anna Karenina*, 'All happy families are alike but an unhappy family is unhappy after its own fashion.' Nothing could be more true of families in which one or more members are dyslexic. By and large the families profiled in this chapter have come to terms with the practical and emotional problems that inevitably accompany dyslexia, in the variety of ways described. They have recognized their problems, faced up to them, and talked them through.

There can be no doubt that where the reality of dyslexia is not confronted the problems are much worse. All those close to the reality of dyslexia – whether they be members of dyslexic families or professionals on the periphery offering advice – will testify to the truth of this statement. Examples of the problems where the reality is either denied or simply ignored are hard to come by since, by definition, they tend to be kept hidden. The following is a compilation of experiences, from a number of families, which provide an impression of the pattern of difficulties that can easily occur inside a dyslexic family.

Invariably, problems are compounded where the father is dyslexic. This is doubly the case where he seeks to deny his dyslexia, a very common experience. Often the denial is driven by the need to create an impression of competence outside the home, especially in a work situation. Inevitably, however, such a denial is reflected back into the home and particularly on to the children.

Where some children are dyslexic and others are not, they can be treated differently. For instance, a dyslexic parent may over-identify and form a more positive relationship with a child who is not dyslexic than with a sibling who is. Then again, a dyslexic parent may present a totally different, perhaps warm, outgoing and friendly, image outside the family compared with inside where resentment and insecurity can be allowed full play. The impact on the dyslexic children can then be imagined. It can be a process of guilt working in two directions, repressed by the parent, but none the less perceived and reflected back, often unconsciously, by the child.

The potential for problems following on from such family dynamics is endless. All who experience dyslexia, whether directly or as a relative, teacher, psychologist or counsellor, will have their own stories to tell. What is remarkable is that in the mass of literature that is now being produced on almost every aspect of an expanding subject, so little is to be found on the family dynamics of dyslexia. Yet it is undeniable that all dyslexic people experience the condition within the context of a family, unless and until they are removed for whatever reason from the family situation.

Nothing can be more important for dyslexics and the larger number of people who relate to them - taken together, as many as 10 per cent of the population - than to have some understanding of how best to live with it. There is probably no other arena more important than the family within which the reality of dyslexia needs to be appreciated and understood.

Chapter 5

Schools

Jason John, brought up in the 1980s in the London borough of Hackney, is an all too typical example of a child who, having failed to be diagnosed as dyslexic and appropriately taught when he was younger, became lost inside the school system.

From when he was at the relatively early age of six to seven – the time when the dyslexic diagnosis should have been made – his parents and teachers both became aware that something was fundamentally wrong with the way he was developing. Yet it was not until he was eleven, just before entering secondary school, that he was discovered to be dyslexic, at the Watford Dyslexia Unit. At that late stage he was found to have a reading age of between five and six.

Jason described how frustrated he had become: 'I feel I'm last in the class and behind all the time,' he said. 'I often get stuck on words but I don't want to ask anyone about it. Sometimes I feel mad but I never let it out. I don't know why. I suppose it's because there is no one really to speak to in school about it. It's just like there's something in my brain that won't click open.'

When he was seven Jason's problems were recognized to the extent that he was put on a remedial accelerated-learning programme, involving one-to-one reading support for two hours a week. As the school's teachers reported, normally children responded positively to this help after six months. However, though Jason was kept on the scheme for two years, he failed to make progress.

Jason's headmaster described the situation in the following terms:

After two years the support was withdrawn because it was felt that we weren't able to solve Jason's particular reading problem. Both the support team and myself felt there was a specific difficulty which required greater support than we were able to give. We've decided to ask for a full psychological assessment, but in the present climate of financial constraints I couldn't say whether we are going to have that report made or not.

Jason is a bright child who joined in activities with enthusiasm when he was younger. He is no longer keen to join in. He will withdraw from particular groups and activities with which he finds difficulty.

If we are having story time he enjoys being part of a group and his recall of stories is better than for most children. His general involvement is excellent. But when it comes to any written form of work or, of course, reading on his own, he withdraws. He finds that sort of activity impossible and he will deploy any form of diversive activity to ensure he doesn't have to be involved. He will ask the teacher if he can do a particular job, ask if he can work in the infants section so that he can be with younger children, and generally withdraw from the class situation rather than continue to face failure.

Jason doesn't misbehave badly in school, but that could be a scenario which might follow. Either he might play truant because he is no longer able to keep up with his peers, or because he is continually facing failure and has no hope of success.

I think Jason is a classic illustration of the type of child who has specific learning difficulties, recognizes that the school has failed him - because we have - and doesn't know who to blame. He feels guilty in his own mind that he is failing and also resents the fact that the school has failed him.

The headmaster's reference to Jason having 'specific learning difficulties' in one sense summarizes both the issue and the problem. There is no consensus and a general lack of knowledge in the schools, certainly primary schools, about dyslexia - whether it actually exists as a definable condition and how it should be tackled. Indeed, part of the problem is the fact that for many educational psychologists and teachers the terms 'dyslexia' and 'specific learning difficulty (Sp LD)' are interchangeable, which only adds to the confusion.

In Jason's case it later emerged that he was indeed suffering from dyslexia and that if appropriate teaching had been available to him he would have made much better progress. Put at its lowest, even if his academic progress had remained slow, his emotional state and outlook would have been much improved. Yet, the fact that his headteacher recognized him to have a 'specific learning difficulty', but did not know how to cope with it, only emphasizes the dilemma. Part of the dilemma is also contained in the absence of agreement in the schools about specific learning difficulty (dyslexia) and what the response to it should be.

This position was reflected in a survey of local education authorities initiated by the British Psychological Society in 1988, and published in 1991. It found that only two in five authorities had formulated a policy on how to deal with dyslexia, or what many preferred to term 'specific learning difficulties', and only a quarter of those had put their policy in writing.

The survey conducted by Professor Peter Pumfrey and Dr Rea Reason of Manchester University, and published in their book *Specific Learning Difficulties (Dyslexia)*, covered 104 local education authorities (the work began prior to the break-up of the Inner London Education Authority) and 882 educational psychologists.

Three-quarters of the councils replied, and of these forty-two (53 per cent) had worked out a policy of some kind. But only twenty-four (30 per cent) had put their policy in writing. In thirteen cases this was in the form of a report to the education committee asking for extra money to spend on such children. The survey found that more and more parents, often supported by dyslexia units, associations and consultants, were seeking help for their children. At the same time more and more teachers were becoming aware of their duty to identify special needs under the 1981 Education Act.

However, the attitude of the psychologists surveyed was revealing. They were asked if they found the terms 'specific learning difficulties' and 'dyslexia' useful in their professional work. Eighty-seven per cent found the former term useful, and 22 per cent thought the two usages were more or less synonymous. But only 30 per cent thought 'dyslexia' was a helpful term. One said: 'Dyslexia sounds like an incurable disease.' Another remarked: 'Dyslexia has become a commercial product and a journalistic victim.'

WHEN DYSLEXIA IS DENIED

Meetings held between the Schools Council, the GCE and CSE examination boards and the British Medical Council at the end of the 1970s failed to agree on a working definition of dyslexia. In 1980 the BMA advised its members that dyslexia was not a medical problem but more the province of the educational psychologist.

Neurologists disagreed, however. As early as 1969 the World Federation of Neurology had defined dyslexia as 'a disorder in children who, despite conventional classroom experience, fail to attain the language skills of reading, writing and spelling commensurate with their intellectual abilities. . . . It is dependent upon fundamental cognitive disabilities which are frequently constitutional in origin.'

Writing in 1981 Dr Macdonald Critchley, a consultant neurologist and an authority in the field, declared: 'I have always insisted that the diagnosis of specific developmental dyslexia is a medical responsibility. This view is not popular among certain educational psychologists, but its truth can scarcely be denied.' He went on to add that dyslexia was genetically determined:

> It is not due to intellectual inadequacy or to lack of socio-cultural opportunity, or to emotional factors, or to any known structural brain defect.
>
> It probably represents a specific maturational defect which tends to lessen as the child grows older, and is capable of considerable improvement, especially when appropriate remedial help is afforded at the earliest opportunity.

Ten years later the authors of the survey already quoted, Professor Pumfrey and Dr Reason, commented: 'Recent advanced work in neurology supports Critchley's comments concerning the neurological integrity of children identified as having specific developmental dyslexia. These findings may, if anything, strengthen the case for neurologists' involvement in assessment and diagnosis.' They added that educational psychologists who still maintained that the cause of dyslexia was relatively unimportant compared with identifying and alleviating the difficulties it brought about revealed 'a questionable certitude. If, as has been suggested, the brain of a dyslexic person is "miswired", it is not a point to be dismissed lightly.'

By the 1990s, therefore, the balance of view was shifting in favour of dyslexia being understood as an identifiable condition whose causes are rooted in inherited genes, as described in Chapter 1, rather than being an 'unidentified flying object of psychology', cited by Pumfrey and Reason as the view of one university professor.

This dispute between neurologists and psychologists is mirrored at another level, between educationalists, and reflected in turn in the classroom. It can be roughly summarized as the *top–down* versus the *bottom–up* approach to the way children learn and absorb information.

Proponents of the top–down theory consider that, in mastering such complex skills as reading, writing and spelling, the most effective procedure is to engage in the activity itself, as a whole. An analogy might be that children learn to swim by swimming, or learn to ride a bike simply by getting on a bike and riding. So, it is claimed, children learn to read by reading. This has been expressed in perhaps its most notorious form by the Canadian educationalist, Frank Smith, who claimed that 'dyslexia is not a medical problem', in his book *Reading* (Cambridge University Press, 1985):

> To learn to read, children need to be helped to read. The issue is as simple and difficult as that . . .
> Dyslexia is a name, not an explanation. Dyslexia means, quite literally, being unable to read. Children who experience difficulty learning to read are frequently called dyslexic, but their difficulty does not arise because they *are* dyslexic, or because they *have* dyslexia; they are dyslexic because they cannot read. To say that dyslexia is a cause of not being able to read is analogous to saying that lameness is a cause of not being able to walk. We were all dyslexic at one stage of our lives and become dyslexic again whenever we are confronted by something that we cannot read. The cure for dyslexia is to read.

This perspective, in effect a denial of dyslexia, not only flies in the face of mounting scientific evidence, but is a product of a top–down approach to education. It is a view that that instruction progresses from the general to the specific. In the case of reading it stresses the importance of meaning, where children begin with stories and poems, after which letter and word recognition skills follow.

While this may empirically be the case with most children, it is emphatically not the case with the dyslexic child. As the British Dyslexia Association's material on the subject puts it:

> The methods generally used in mainstream schools for children beginning to learn to read are those based on the 'whole word' approach.
> While the majority of children learn very successfully in this way, the dyslexic child does not. S/he fails to learn new words and even

words once learnt are quickly forgotten. While some children successfully learn to 'read from reading' dyslexic children, along with many others, do not learn in this way. They need to be taught decoding skills.

Dyslexic children seem to have a very poor memory capacity for words. This is why so many of them cannot learn to read efficiently by the 'whole word' or 'look and say' approach. The methods favoured by teachers working with dyslexic children are based on a structured language programme which teaches sound/letter relationships, blending of letters, syllable division, spelling rules and choices, study skills and organization. The dyslexic child responds best to an alphabetic approach to learning whereby s/he is taught in a systematic and cumulative way each letter of the alphabet for sound, name and written shape. The letters are gradually built into syllables, then words, then phrases and sentences and finally prose for both reading and spelling.

The method is multi-sensory, that is learning by all pathways – visual, auditory, spoken, and kinaesthetic. This can be an exciting approach for both teacher and learner.

In addition a joined style of writing should be taught as soon as the child is expected to write anything down. There is no evidence to support the contention that this is too large a step for young children and that print script is more appropriate at this stage. Indeed, all the evidence shows that a joined style of writing can aid spelling. In particular flowing letter-strings should be encouraged.

Later the dyslexic child will need to be taught specific aspects of the English language which s/he will not pick up from reading: information about vowels, spelling choices and probabilities, spelling rules, prefixes, suffixes, alphabet and dictionary skills. . . .

What all this points to is an emphasis for dyslexic children on a *bottom–up* approach to teaching, certainly so far as reading, writing and spelling are concerned. There are, of course, many possible variations on the advice just quoted, with due attention being given to the individual needs of each child. But as Pumfrey and Reason conclude in their survey: 'Currently an individualised multisensory approach in which phonics play a large part is favoured by the majority of the specialist organisations. Such approaches have a distinctly *bottom–up* flavour.'

The trouble is that mainstream schools tend to deploy what they generally regard as a 'normal' top–down approach when teaching children to read. This is the environment within which most dyslexic children, whether they have been identified as dyslexic or not, have to survive. In it the leading role is given first to overall meaning, and only secondly to strategies that ensure the kind of accuracy of perception listed above. That this invariably leaves the dyslexic child stranded, bewildered and very soon alienated is a matter of fulsome testimony by dyslexic children and adults, as seen in previous chapters.

Awareness of dyslexia is spreading rapidly, but at the same time there is resistance on the part of some local education authorities and many teachers to its being defined as a problem. There are many reasons for this. In the first place, as has been seen, the cause of dyslexia is a complex, not to say controversial, matter, still subject to extensive research.

It is further complicated, however, in at least three further specific ways. First, since every person is an individual every dyslexic person will experience dyslexia in an individual way. It is difficult, if not impossible, therefore, to disentangle reading and writing skills from the emotional and personality background of a person. For instance, problems can arise from parents who see their child having difficulty and becoming anxious, perhaps over-anxious. This in turn can make the child anxious and compound the difficulties.

Secondly, the dyslexia issue, partly because of its controversial background, is inevitably caught up with the politics of local education policy and funding. Resources are finite and there are many calls on the funds of local education authorities and schools. There is undoubtedly a widespread feeling amongst some teachers, directors of education and others directly involved, that people agitating on behalf of dyslexic children are, by definition, middle class and articulate and therefore likely to achieve a disproportionate share of scarce resources.

Lastly, and most problematically, dyslexia tends to be identified with failure. Children found to be dyslexic are more often than not discovered as a result of 'failing' at school in the sense of not fulfilling the expectations of their parents and teachers. What is often not taken into account is that the parents and teachers can feel that they have failed themselves. Often they can feel that, for some inexplicable reason, they have been unable to communicate with the child in question and thereby failed to pass on basic skills with which other apparently similar children find little difficulty. A sense of guilt can then possess a teacher, who may in turn look for alternative explanations – usually in the upbringing and background of the child.

Alternatively, and perhaps more commonly, such feelings can simply be suppressed, which in many ways is a worse scenario. Certainly this explanation can lie behind the vehemence with which arguments over dyslexia are often conducted.

Any combination of these reasons can even lead to a straightforward denial of dyslexia. For instance, in the early 1990s one comprehensive school in England, beset by parents anxious about the reading and writing abilities of their children, produced a policy statement declaring emphatically and unambiguously the following two points:

> *A definition of dyslexia will not help a child. A definition of dyslexia will not help a teacher to help a child.*

It went on to say:

> Some parents may be surprised by these assertions. Others will feel relieved that any pressure to pursue this definition because others have done so has been removed. Extra lessons at the Dyslexia Institute or private tuition by dyslexia trained tutors is likely to inhibit the success of the programmes and strategies promoted by the school . . .
> Literacy problems arise from a complicated interaction of factors. To attempt to quantify their exact relationship would be impossible. Furthermore, we do come across many situations where we do not know the exact cause, but that doesn't prevent us from seeking a satisfactory solution. The problem with the term dyslexia is that by being accepted as a reason it can directly impede the solution and sometimes mask identification of real reasons . . .

As has been said, such a straightforward denial of dyslexia as a genetically based constitutional condition flies in the face of mounting, scientifically based evidence. In the policy declaration just quoted there is an attempt to support the denial with the claim that children can be harmed by being 'labelled' dyslexic: 'Owning a label often leads to accepting the problem and unconsciously losing the belief that a solution is possible,' the paper states.

Again, however, this flies against the weight of evidence. Without exception the dyslexic people interviewed in this book indicated how much they were helped in coming to terms with their condition simply by understanding there was an explanation, a cause. This is fully documented throughout the literature on dyslexia, now running to thousands of titles. In his study *Dyslexia:*

The Pattern of Difficulties Professor Tim Miles devotes a chapter to the issue. He records how the hundreds of dyslexic people, mainly children, he has diagnosed have invariably achieved enormous relief and enhanced self-confidence at discovering there was indeed a label which could describe their problem:

> Secret fears that they were stupid, or even mad, were regularly found among my subjects, and it was sometimes possible to bring these fears into the open. For example, it transpired that one 12-year-old boy had earlier been worried that he was, in his words, a 'nut-case', and when his mother described how he and some slower children had been 'loaded' together (that is, put in the same 'band' at school) he commented 'Some *were* nut-cases' . . .

And as another leading authority in the field of dyslexia studies, Dr Macdonald Critchley, put it, in his book *The Dyslexic Child*:

> Once a child is diagnosed as being the victim of a genuine inherent disability and not a naughty, stupid, lazy or neurotic youngster, his self-respect is immediately enhanced and any bad behaviour he may have shown comes to an end, without any intervention on the part of child psychiatry.

Returning to the school policy statement quoted above: what it reveals is teachers trying to come to terms with children in their care experiencing obvious difficulties, but at the same time refusing to acknowledge the reasons for the problems. Often the distinction is a subtle one, but none the less crucial. Such teachers often allow the presence of special needs in relation to literacy, but deny their definition in terms of dyslexia or are simply unaware of the condition. Sometimes they resort to the phrase 'specific learning difficulty', as was the case with Jason John's headmaster quoted near the beginning of this chapter. It may be argued that as this amounts to much the same thing the distinction does not matter. And, indeed, that is the view of many professionals in the field.

Yet this remains a denial of dyslexia as a congenital, genetically inherited condition. The result is twofold. First, far from harming children, it denies children the possibility of release from guilt and responsibility that the 'label' dyslexia invariably brings. And, secondly, the failure to appreciate fully the nature of the problem means that teachers tend not to appreciate the impact of dyslexia on children as *whole* emotional persons, rather than simply as it affects their learning difficulties at school.

SURVIVING DESPITE THE SYSTEM

As has already been emphasized, no dyslexic person is exactly like another. This is part of the problem of recognizing and ameliorating the condition within the mainstream school system. It can be argued, however, that dyslexic children fall into broadly three categories.

First there are a minority who are so severely dyslexic that there is no mistaking that something is wrong. Their fate depends on whether their condition is recognized to be what it is. With such children, who usually display a pattern of emotional problems as well as the classic signs of dyslexia, there is usually no effective option but for them to be cared for outside the mainstream school system. The lucky ones reside within a local education authority that is prepared to make a Statement under the 1981 Education Act delineating their special needs, and as a result send them to a special school dedicated to teaching dyslexic children.

More often than not, and for understandable if misguided reasons, LEAs are reluctant to take such a step, usually because of the financial implications. Generally, parents have to fight their cause and often make great financial sacrifices themselves to ensure their children are properly looked after. Invariably it is the parents who are most determined, articulate and financially well-off who win through. In this, as in many other areas of their lives, dyslexic children spin through a lottery.

Where they are not discovered, usually as a result of having unaware teachers and inarticulate parents, severely dyslexic children tend to be identified as simply backward, emotionally disturbed, or even retarded, and left to languish on the edge of the generally overstretched education system.

The second category of dyslexic children is very difficult to quantify since they are highly likely to remain forever unidentified. It is one of the great misconceptions in the debate around dyslexia that dyslexic children are invariably of at least average and usually above-average intelligence. Yet this is simply a reflection of the fact that such children can be more easily seen to be failing to achieve what would generally be expected. All the available research indicates that dyslexia occurs in people of every kind of social and cultural background and of every level of intelligence. With dyslexic children of relatively low intelligence their fate usually is to be doubly disadvantaged, to be identified not just as backward and deposited for ever in the remedial section of school, but to be labelled educationally subnormal as well.

The third category of dyslexic children, and undoubtedly the most numerous, are those who fall within a spectrum of severity between the first two types. They may be exceptionally bright children who tend to be able to cope by themselves and are seen by their teachers and peers as in some ways odd, especially in terms of social interaction, but otherwise 'normal'. Though they are generally average in their academic performance, typically however they tend to experience problems around the age of thirteen or fourteen especially in organizing and structuring work such as essay writing. They may have managed up to that point, but suddenly the workload can become too much for them to deliver. Moreover, although these children are of generally average or slightly above-average intelligence and ability, if that ability is to be expressed it tends to rely on the intervention of supportive, articulate parents. It is the parents who struggle against an inert, often hostile education system to ensure that their children have adequate help to enable them to survive within the mainstream school.

One such example is James Moran. No story is really typical. In James's case he was fortunate to have particularly educated and articulate parents. His father is a consultant physician. His mother is a teacher who, as a result of her experiences with the three of her four children who are dyslexic, has trained in dyslexic teaching techniques. None the less, James's story is instructive in at least two respects. First, it is revealing of the attitudes that can be encountered within the mainstream school system. Secondly, it is an example of how it is possible for a dyslexic child to survive, despite the system.

When James was nine years old his parents became concerned at his lack of progress. As his mother, Carolyn, put it:

> He could barely write a sentence, and when he read aloud he sounded like a Dalek out of Dr Who. On visits to parents' evenings at the primary school we were told 'it would come'. It didn't, and eventually in desperation I taught him at home for a term.
>
> During that time he was seen by an independent educational psychologist who pronounced him to be intelligent (IQ 120) and dyslexic. In our ignorance, we thought our problems were over.

Since there were no trained dyslexia teachers available in James's school or on the county support team, a tutor qualified in multisensory, structured methods of teaching was found and James went for private lessons, twice a week. These continued for four years, during which time James's parents also paid for him to attend an independent school where they felt he would receive closer, more sympathetic, individual attention. 'By the time he was twelve he was coping at school, though not, we felt, reaching his full potential,' said Carolyn Moran. 'Still, we felt relieved, thinking the worst was over.'

When James was fourteen and ready to begin GCSE course work, it was decided that he could manage in the neighbourhood state comprehensive school. By now he had come to grips with many of his literacy problems. His spelling was still weak, and his sentences rambled, largely because of the efforts he had to put into the mechanics of writing and forming letters, which distracted him from the overall content of what he was trying to say. However, with his lap-top word processor his use of vocabulary was much improved and his ideas came across in a more logical sequence. Even without its built-in spellcheck the machine was plainly a key to unlock James's powers of expression. As Carolyn Moran put it:

After years of struggle, his ability was beginning to emerge.

Our next move was to ask the English department at the school to consider moving him up a set. At the start he had been placed in a low-ability group which messed about and did not appear to be motivated. We asked the school to put him in a group that matched his IQ so that the lessons would be more stimulating. Initially, the school stalled, but we persisted and they agreed to review the situation. James was placed in a room by himself, handed a poem and given an hour to answer questions on it, using his Z88. On the basis of these results they agreed to try him in a set where he could obtain a grade of C or higher at GCSE. It was up to him to prove he could do it.

We visited the school several times to discuss aspects of James's difficulties. Everybody was extremely pleasant but nobody really understood why he needed the lap-top computer. I suspect James had to spend an hour doing the poem because they thought we had done the previous word-processed work for him, which of course we hadn't. Having seen his poor handwritten work, I think his teachers didn't believe he was capable of much better. One teacher told James during a lesson in which he was using his lap-top, 'I don't know why you use that thing. You won't be allowed it for GCSE exams.'

At this stage James's parents decided to have him independently assessed once more, in an effort to persuade the examination boards to allow him extra time and use of his word processor when sitting his GCSEs. As his mother put it:

> He had great difficulty planning and organizing his work and his written language expression and spelling were still significantly below par. His needs had to be reviewed for exam concessions.
>
> Our county makes minimal provision for dyslexic pupils and in addition the attitudes of the county educational psychologists vary widely towards dyslexia. Moreover, parents cannot choose which LEA educational psychologist performs the assessment. If he or she happens to be unsympathetic or sceptical about dyslexia, time is wasted. For these reasons we opted to pay to have James assessed by the Dyslexia Institute. The findings confirmed his special needs and we were given a lengthy report and a concessionary certificate requesting that the exam boards take his difficulties into account. It was recommended that he be allowed extra time and use of a word processor to compensate for his poor fine motor co-ordination and to help him express his ideas more coherently.

On receipt of the report the school asked the parents to see their own LEA educational psychologist before submitting it to the examination boards. Carolyn Moran recalls that it was a tense meeting. 'From the moment he entered the room, the psychologist radiated aggression,' she said.

> Firstly, he informed us that he did not accept the Dyslexia Institute's report and would have to run his own tests on James before deciding whether exam concessions were allowable. He stated that James must not be given an unfair advantage – a worthy sentiment which would have been laughable had it not been so heartbreaking in its ignorance.
>
> He said that use of a word processor was out of the question. To qualify for that you would have to be incapacitated and in a wheelchair. He would decide himself whether James had learning difficulties. In his opinion the Dyslexia Institute often erroneously identified children as dyslexic because much of its income came from teaching them. Yet the fact that James had never been taught by one of the institute's tutors seemed to escape him.

Momentarily, James's parents were stunned by this interview. But they decided to press on. 'We did not feel inclined to return to square one and begin arguing over again about whether James was really dyslexic,' said Carolyn Moran.

> To say that extra time would give James an 'unfair advantage' was ridiculous. We had lived with his difficulties and watched his

struggles for seven years and we knew the difference that proper structured help had made to him. His only chance of getting the grades which would reflect his ability was to be permitted the use of his Z88. If he had to handwrite his papers he would do badly, because for him writing and spelling are not automatic processes. He just can't do them and simultaneously express ideas in an able and coherent fashion. Extra time on its own does not solve the problem.

So she contacted James's two examination boards, the Midlands Examining Group and the Southern Examining Group, and discovered that the report from the Dyslexia Institute, conducted as it had been by a qualified psychologist, was perfectly acceptable. As a result the LEA psychologist's insistence that he conduct his own assessment was ignored and James's case was submitted on the basis of the institute's report alone.

The judgement that came back was that James was to be refused the word processor, but allowed 25 per cent extra time to compensate for his slow handwriting speed. An undertaking was made that his spelling would not be penalized and so spelling concessions were unnecessary.

James's parents sought a second opinion on the word processor. On the basis of a second psychologist's report James was granted use of his lap-top computer in his History exam. His parents confirmed once more with the boards that spelling concessions were not needed.

However, shortly after the examinations were under way they heard from the school that the Midlands Examining Group Board had decided to penalize spelling after all. They then had three options: do nothing and allow James to be penalized like everyone else; inform the board of his dyslexia so that the individual examiner could bear it in mind and decide whether to make allowances or not; or apply for James's spelling errors to be ignored but have his exam certificates endorsed.

'We opted for the last choice,' said Carolyn Moran.

James has never made a secret of his dyslexia, and in the real world of jobs it is perfectly acceptable to use spellcheckers and lap-tops to overcome difficulties. We thought he should be given every chance to obtain the best grades he could. At any interviews in the future he would be able to explain about his dyslexic problems and also show how he had had the character and determination to overcome them.

Then there was another setback. The Southern Examining Group Board, in another perverse, last-minute reversal of attitude, decided to take off marks for poor spelling. The decision was that if James wanted his spelling errors discounted he would have to forgo his extra time. As his Southern Examining Group subjects were Maths and Technology, where spelling is less high-profile, it was decided to choose the extra time.

Carolyn Moran commented:

> In these apparently last-minute decisions by the examination boards we encountered yet again a feature that has struck us throughout James's school career, lack of understanding from institutions.
>
> Extra time and spelling concessions should not be an either/or. Dyslexics frequently write laboriously and have difficulty expressing their ideas sequentially. They take much longer than their peers to plan work and read exam questions.
>
> That is why extra time is useful. It is much less helpful as a means to check spelling, as often dyslexic people cannot see what is wrong with a word, however hard they look. James's weak skills in spelling will dog him all his life, through no lack of effort on his part. Why cannot this be taken into account, or a spellchecker permitted to help his deficiency?

Lack of understanding on the part of institutions extended in James's case to his school. While in most other respects the school was supportive, it proved inflexible where the curriculum was concerned. Some time before he sat his GCSEs James's parents decided that it would be counterproductive for him to continue with French. They wrote to the school asking for him to cease studying the subject, giving four reasons:

1. The educational psychologists who had submitted reports recommended it.
2. James's dyslexic problem meant that there was no hope of his achieving a meaningful grade. His particular cluster of deficits meant that he could neither retain French by ear nor remember it visually.
3. His performance within the French class was at such a low level that his residual self-esteem was being undermined by this subject more than any other. It was damaging for him to continue with a subject where he had little chance of success.
4. The session could be more usefully devoted to other things, for instance catching up with course work in other subjects.

The school refused the request, the headmaster saying in a letter: 'I have to make the difficult judgement as to the overall benefit of the institution . . . I am not prepared to allow the precedent that would be created by the course you propose.' In a further letter he added: 'The thrust of the National Curriculum and of school curricular policy is that subjects such as French can and must be made accessible to all pupils.'

James's parents appealed to the school governors against the headmaster's decision, which had been supported by the county educational psychologist. Obtaining a further report from their independent psychologist, and also their general practitioner, they summarized their case in the following terms:

> The issue boils down to the convenience of the school against the welfare of an individual pupil. . . . In a rigid curriculum there has to be some degree of flexibility to meet the needs of a dyslexic pupil such as James. It seems clear that the school is not 'using its best endeavours' to meet this pupil's needs, but rather putting its own convenience first.

In the event the appeal was upheld. For the last two terms before he sat his GCSEs James was able to drop French. In the exams he passed with eight grades: a B in Drama; Cs in English Language and Literature, Double Science, Maths and Technology; and a D in History. These were enough for him to make it into the sixth form to study Social Biology, Sociology and Theatre Studies.

Reflecting on the years of getting James to this point Carolyn Moran said:

> Walking through treacle is the most apt way to describe our experiences with a dyslexic child in the education system. It has been a marathon effort to convince the authorities that James has a genuine, underlying problem which prevents him reaching his potential. We have often been told by teachers 'but there are others far worse in the class'. Surely that is not the point. Every pupil should have the chance to do his or her personal best, whatever that may be.
>
> James's level of frustration has at times been considerable and our energy nearly exhausted. No one tells parents of dyslexic children that the quality they need most of all is stamina if they want to see their offspring through the school years successfully. On numerous occasions we have almost thrown in the towel, and I am a dyslexic tutor myself. If we feel like this, what is it like for others who know less about this very specialist area of disability?

se, easy to criticize. Teachers in mainstream schools
able problems. Invariably they are overstretched in
cla___ so full of children that it is difficult to give those without special problems the attention they deserve, let alone those with
disabilities such as dyslexia. Usually they have not been trained in
recognizing or coping with dyslexic children.

Yet there can be no doubt that most dyslexic children have to
make their way through mainstream schools. And for the majority
of moderately dyslexic children they would not wish it otherwise.
The alternative, of attending a dedicated special school, even if
within reach financially, has built-in disadvantages. Few children
enjoy being singled out as 'different'. Attending a special school
inevitably entails this kind of identification and, in any event, most
children are better off based at home with their families.

This, too, is the view of most professional advisers in the education field. Certainly, it was emphasized in the 1981 Education Act
that as far as possible children with special needs should be integrated within the mainstream school setting, rather than be treated
separately. However, a reading of this book, and especially the
present chapter, provides ample evidence of how far we have to
travel in terms of attitudes and resources before dyslexic children
can be said to be dealt with adequately within the mainstream
school system.

An initial problem is one of identification. The traditional
approach to assessment for dyslexia – screening by an elaborate
series of psychological tests – has many limitations. To begin with
they are immensely time-consuming. Moreover, they are far from
precise. They comprise a selection of factors, including verbal and
non-verbal reasoning, comprehension and vocabulary, which are
all affected by previous learning and experience.

Even where local education authorities allow a screening process,
more often than not they wait until a child has reached eight years
or more. This can mean that where such a child is found to be
dyslexic he or she has already experienced at least three years of
failure.

Another dilemma is that the identification procedures tend to
focus on the more able children. With them the gap between intelligence and ability in reading and writing attainment more clearly

stands out. On the other hand, with less intelligent children the discrepancy is not so obvious and so they tend to go unrecognized.

Equally, dyslexic children of above average intelligence and ability often appear to be progressing satisfactorily through school and as a result tend to go unrecognized as well. Janet Tod, a researcher into dyslexia who has drawn attention to these limitations of the traditional testing methods, commented:

> Without appropriate help such children are likely to enter on the downward spiral of poorer performance on tasks relating to written language, greater frustration in school work, lower levels of measured IQ (since the tests at higher age levels tend to be more language dependent) and, paradoxically, less likelihood of being identified as dyslexic because the discrepancy between IQ score and attainment is less pronounced!

Another issue, on the face of it a simple concern but none the less highlighted by Janet Tod, is that dyslexia testing usually takes place in an artificial, sometimes stressful environment and atmosphere – the interview room of an educational psychologist. As she says, 'The procedure and task demands tend to be divorced from the actual curricular demands which the pupil faces every day. It is as if the testing takes place in an enclosed capsule. The danger is that all too frequently the assessment and recommendations do not match the *pupil-in-school problem*.'

Janet Tod is Research Co-ordinator of the Dyslexia Project based at the Harris City Technology College in London. Funded by the Department for Education, it has as its aim to develop and evaluate approaches to dyslexia in mainstream schools. The first stage has been to compare traditional assessment procedures, whose limitations have been discussed above, with an alternative approach centred around the attainment targets in the English curriculum specified by the 1988 Education Reform Act. These are *Speaking and Listening, Reading, Writing, Presentation and Handwriting*. The research, which began in late 1990, hinges around the reasonable assumption that the attainment of dyslexic children in the written aspects of English will be poorer than their performance in *Speaking and Listening*. Early indications are hopeful. They show that National Curriculum classroom-based assessment can serve to differentiate dyslexic pupils.

The National Curriculum English tests were carried out on a group of ordinary secondary school children and compared with a group already identified as dyslexic. They revealed, as would be expected, that the dyslexic children responded well to the *Speaking and Listening* part of the test, and most of them had learnt to cope with reading – that is to say, in Janet Tod's words, they had 'cracked the code'. When it came to the other parts of the test – *Writing* and *Presentation and Handwriting* – however, they were found to be functioning significantly below the levels of the other group, by a factor of two on the scores deployed. As Janet Tod commented:

> This is a significant difference. And crucially National Curriculum tests will be applied uniformly and evenly across the country. This means there is scope for all teachers to identify the dyslexic children in their classrooms.
>
> The dyslexic child will not then be dependent upon vociferous parental demands, well above average ability or residence within the boundaries of a particular local education authority in order to obtain an assessment of oral and written language.
>
> Whilst acknowledging the contribution which specialist teaching has made to the education of dyslexic pupils the challenge now is to determine the extent to which provision for such children can be delivered in an integrated setting.

The challenge, too, is to extend the research, using National Curriculum English testing, to see how far dyslexic children can be identified at primary school, when they are between five and seven. Early indications are that here testing on *Speaking and Listening* and seeing how it compares with *Reading* and *Writing* is less reliable in picking out the dyslexic child.

However, Janet Tod believes that as the tests become more familiar to teachers, and as their awareness of dyslexia grows, there should be scope for much greater accuracy in identifying dyslexic children early in their school careers. If this is followed on a wide scale there is a chance that at last the needs of the mass of dyslexic children within mainstream schools will be identified. Such recognition is an essential preliminary to the needs of dyslexic children in schools being met.

Chapter 6

Extraordinary, Ordinary People

> When asked what he felt was the worst thing a school could do to
> a dyslexic, he answered immediately, 'Taking all their confidence
> away.' . . . He himself describes his special school provision in terms
> of being saved from life as a thug.

Janice Edwards, who is preparing a study entitled *The Scars of
Dyslexia*, made these comments about an eleven-year-old boy,
John Saines, who came into her care at Brickwell House Special
School near Rye in East Sussex. It is one of the first of many that
have grown up to deal with the needs of severely dyslexic children,
especially since the 1981 Education Act.

There is little doubt that for some severely dyslexic children there
is no option but for them to be educated away from home in a
special school where appropriate and concentrated attention can
be given to their problems. However, for financial reasons alone,
this can only apply to a minority of children. As was seen in the
previous chapter most dyslexic children have to be helped within
the conventional school system.

The problem is that as things stand there is not the knowledge,
the will or imagination to enable this to happen effectively on the
scale that is required. The consequences of neglect, however, can
be profound.

John Saines's story is a case in point, and a warning. He was fortunate to be identified as a dyslexic in London early on in his school
career, when he was just under seven. His mother was very supportive, particularly since she is dyslexic herself. He was lucky, as well,
to be able to take refuge in sporting achievement. At the same

time, however, he was faced with a succession of teachers who were bewildered and frustrated by his problems and who had little idea how to cope with them.

After long battles with a reluctant Inner London Education Authority John's parents finally managed to persuade them to fund him to board at Brickwall House Special School. This is how Janice Edwards described what happened when he first appeared there, in her class of eight children: 'He was a loud eleven-year-old with slightly rough manners, an infectious grin and a strong but soft-voiced cockney accent. He described his previous schools with great confidence: "I 'ated the first, but the second was a great laugh. Didn't learn nothin' though."' The subject that day was Geography and a lesson that consisted of copious coloured diagrams and short facts about coastal erosion, printed on the white board in front of the class. 'John copied a whole board of writing and diagrams faster than I could write,' Janice Edwards recalled.

> Meanwhile, the rest of the children were struggling, looking at the diagrams and generally reading the material through as they were told.
>
> But John's work was perfectly copied, very rare for a dyslexic. I thought to myself, 'Why is he here?' Then I asked him to read it to me on his own and he couldn't decipher a word. He had copied it symbol by symbol, eye to paper without being able to process a word. I asked him how he did it and he said his last teacher used to rap him over the knuckles if he wasn't fast enough, or he'd lose his break and lunch times copying up. So he developed speed. It took me a long time to cure him of non-reading compulsive copying.

When John entered Brickwall House School, at eleven years nine months old, he had a reading age of seven years two months and a spelling age of six years nine months. His IQ, on the Wechsler Intelligence Scale for Children, was 134 for verbal skills and 117 for general performance. The first four years of his formal education had been at a private prep school, followed by a state primary school in London where he stayed two and a half years.

'I used to hate most of the kids,' he told Janice Edwards about his prep school.

> It was a private school and I hated it because all the kids there were bloody clever and I was stupid. They all went on to pass their eleven plus and I couldn't even read the bloody questions.
>
> The teachers I really hated. One of them hit me with the thick end of a broom, right across the side of the head. I had a whacking great

bruise on one side, and a long, thin bruise right across the back of my head. I never told my mum. I used to keep it quiet. I don't think the teacher meant to hit me as hard as she did. I was about six or seven at the time. She was the needlework teacher. You can imagine how needlework and me got on!

There was another teacher who used to hit me over the knuckles very hard with a ruler every time I messed about. I used to throw things around, and skive off work. The feeling went in my knuckles eventually, you get used to it. Mind you, from what I can make out I was a right sod. That teacher once hit me really hard. She asked me to do a piece of work and I just couldn't. She said I was stupid. I said if she was so bleedin' clever let her do it herself. So she hit me. I was always saying things like that. I used to spend all day standing by her desk.

He was teased and bullied by other children at the school, and eventually asked to leave because it was judged he wouldn't pass the eleven-plus examination. Looking back on the period, when he was fourteen years old, he commented, 'It's as simple as this. If you get the mick taken out of you twenty-four hours a day you go crackers.'

When he moved to a state primary school there was some recognition of his problems and some special help given, but it was woefully inadequate. His school reports state that he had remedial help every afternoon. In fact, most of these times John remembers truanting: 'We never used to turn up after lunch in the afternoons,' he said.

No one used to bother. We used to muck about in the yard with a load of cardboard boxes.

The headmaster used to take me and three or four other boys for five minutes' extra reading in the corridor. Then he could say to our parents he was giving us special remedial help. It really used to pee me off. I read *Roderick the Red* six times in two years. I chose it because it was the easiest book in the school. I knew it off by heart in the end. The teacher didn't give a toss. When I finished it she used to make me start it again. She had the worst class in the school and was straight out of college. I had her for all my time there. Still, we were all thick and stupid together. It was a great laugh.

He remembers having a running vendetta with the staff. 'I got my own back, though, it was only fair,' he said. 'Once I sneaked in and blocked the staff loos. I remember feeling really chuffed. They was all women. I couldn't see them using the men's.'

For a while John was taken out of the school once a week to be taught for an hour in a special remedial unit. This he remembered as being spectacularly ineffective: 'It was with this American woman, a right stupid cow,' he said. 'She used to freak me out, making me do exercises like lie on the floor face down and pull myself along with my fingers to help my writing muscles. The best thing was that afterwards my mum and me had Cornish pasties in a pie shop, as a special treat.'

Towards the end of his time in primary school a psychological report, strongly recommending a residential placement, commented:

> John is a likeable boy and gets on well with adults. He has a lot of energy and determination and good intelligence but is very quick to avoid 'the failure situation'. I can only conclude that a large comprehensive will swallow John and this will only strengthen his tendency to withdraw from a failure situation instead of persisting.

At Brickwall House Special School John made rapid progress. His reading age advanced by two and a half years in his first year. Eventually he took five CSEs and three O levels. A notable achievement was an above-average grade 3 in the CSE English Language paper. He became a prolific potter at the school, excelled at sport, entered the Duke of Edinburgh Awards scheme, and became head boy.

His tutor, Janice Edwards, emphasized that when he arrived at Brickwall House it was academic confidence about his school work that was lacking rather than confidence in other ways. 'He was actually rather an extrovert, with a terrific sense of humour and great wit and charm,' she recalled.

> He had a very strong character, tending to be the daring one, the life and soul of the party. That is probably one of the reasons he got into trouble with some teachers. That warm side to him rapidly disappeared, however, in stiff classroom situations.
> When he first came to Brickwall he could be quite difficult to pin down to read, spell or concentrate, even in an individual situation. He was a master at avoidance techniques, distraction strategies and verbal side-tracking from the task in hand. Every lesson involved negotiation. I had to coax, converse and listen to his concerns. We had to have some laughter and a bit of a power struggle before he could calm down and bring himself to read or work.
> It was only really by giving him a lot of choice over tasks, and making a huge effort to provide some variety, language games,

interesting subject matter, and look at things from his point of view whilst pushing the reading and spelling patterns I wanted to get across that we got anywhere.

It seemed as though books were poison to him, and I now put that down to the appalling treatment he received from earlier teachers. At the time it felt like he almost had a phobia about books and needed to be desensitized to them.

Throughout his time at the school John continually had to overcome negative feelings and a lack of self-confidence about his academic attainment. Janice Edwards continued:

When he was fifteen we had long individual discussions, involving teachers and parents and also the games staff, about how John had to feel exceptionally liked before he would co-operate or work for any teacher.

This manifested itself even on the games field, where he was an all-round brilliant performer. We had a protracted discussion about his unwillingness to participate unless he felt he would win. As captain of the football team he was heavily criticized on one occasion for giving up when the opposing team scored rapid goals early on. John gave up trying and the whole team lost heart.

The early stages were always crucial with John, and he found it difficult to rally and fight back once he felt he had slid down. I recall going through his school reports with him as his tutor. He had received the usual batch of As for effort and Cs for achievement. He looked less than elated and I asked him what was wrong.

'It's always the bloody same,' he replied. 'It really guts me off. *Tries hard but gets nowhere*, that's what it means! I wish just once I could get it the other way round for something in school, saying I didn't put meself out but did well anyway. Just once! Like all those other buggers! It ain't fair!'

After he left Brickwall House John went into the building trade and carved out a successful career. Shortly before he left he declared: 'If I hadn't come here I'd have been a skinhead or a Mohican. Worse than that, probably, and I'd have left home by now. All the crowd I used to hang around with were really bad.'

DYSLEXIA AND CRIME

Recounting John Saines's story is one way of illustrating what a full reading of this book should make obvious: that the emotional problems commonly associated with dyslexia – frustration, rejection, inadequacy, poor self-confidence and low self-esteem – can easily underpin deviant behaviour and even lead on to crime. In Chapter 2 we saw in the case of Stephen Bonfield how, but for the sensitive intervention of his special needs teacher at a critical moment, he might have become seriously depressed and alienated in his early teens. The child psychologist, Dr Macdonald Critchley, drew attention to this many years ago in his book *The Dyslexic Child*:

> There may be an aggressive type of reaction from dyslexia which may show itself in a variety of ways, among them temper tantrums, destructiveness, and fighting. Alternatively, there may be day dreaming and playing dumb – the child so to speak retreating into himself.
>
> It is, in fact, possible to meet any of the common manifestations of emotional disturbances, for example, neurosis, stammer, sleep walking, and there are various physical symptoms such as vomiting and recurrent abdominal pain for which no physical cause can be found.
>
> As the child gets older it is to be expected that the behaviour disorders will take a more unsocial or anti-social form. Truancy is rather a phenomenon of secondary school age and much of the same applies to stealing, pathological lying and the drift into the more destructive gang activities. Deep emotional disturbances, quite severe depression, fantasy building and other neurotic manifestations, though apparently not very common, are nevertheless a possibility. . . . The ease with which dyslexic teenagers slip into crime demands serious notice.

One such teenager was Ian May, who began a criminal career with petty theft which led on to much more serious offences. These landed him in prison, eventually Full Sutton High Security Prison near York, serving a six-year sentence. It was there, after three years and when he was twenty-five years old, that Ian discovered he was dyslexic. He was taking an external degree with Leeds University when his tutor saw he was having problems and called in a specialist.

Ian was brought up in Scarborough and remembers having difficulties from his earliest days: 'There was a lot of pressure at home to do well at school,' he said.

> My two sisters did well at school. Both my mother and father have a lot of qualifications. They didn't believe I was thick, they were just convinced I was lazy, especially compared with my sisters.
>
> It made life very uncomfortable because even when I did try to do the school work I just wasn't able to do it. What would take

other kids half an hour to do their work would take me four or five hours. I became so frustrated trying to do it and not being able to that it slowed me down even more and I made more mistakes.

It wound my mother up a lot and it gave me a bad opinion about myself. The other kids at school were convinced I was stupid. The teachers were convinced I was lazy. Nobody said there's a problem here, maybe it's dyslexia. I was tested for other reading and writing difficulties, but nobody came up with any answers other than 'he's just bone idle'.

Looking back it makes me angry because either dyslexia was not known about or nobody made an effort. If I'd found out when I was six or seven that I was dyslexic things could have been done to help me learn. Because nothing was done I went through life with a very low impression of myself. I couldn't say, of course, that if I had been helped I wouldn't have ended up in prison. But it would not be for the reasons I'm here now.

As it was I was set apart from other people. By the time I got into secondary school I was a real loner. I couldn't fit in with any of the different groups of people at school. I didn't fit in with the top classes because my work just wasn't good enough. So I ended up in the remedial classes. But I didn't fit in with the kids there either. I'd come from a middle-class background and had middle-class ideas. The kids in the remedial groups had working-class ideas so there was a conflict there.

I was never any good at things like sport. So there was no area where I could be better than anybody else, and that seemed necessary in a school where everything was competitive. I ended up getting bullied a good deal, especially at the beginning. Towards the end it wasn't so bad, but mainly because I was avoiding situations. I would skip off school and go into town and things like that.

The only way I could see to make friends was to buy things to pass round, especially cigarettes. I was buying friends, but how was I to get the money to buy the cigarettes? I could think of no legitimate way so I ended up burgling houses and using the money from that to buy friends. It started me on a downward spiral. All that happened was that the more I spent on people the more I had to rob to carry on doing it.

In the early 1980s Jill Hutchings, a London probation officer, became convinced that dyslexia was a background reason for many of her clients ending up in prison. The relationship between criminal behaviour and illiteracy or semi-literacy was already well established. For instance, the Home Office estimated that, on the basis of reception testing, more than 20 per cent of those in prison, youth custody centres or detention centres had a reading age of less than ten years. A 1981 study by the Inner London Probation Service of clients engaged in adventure training activities revealed that a quarter of the sample had some kind of literacy problem, with more than 10 per cent totally illiterate.

The probability is that such figures seriously underestimate the scale of the problem. As Jill Hutchings remarked, 'My own experience as a probation officer in East Sussex and London suggests that many clients complete their period of probation without any effort being made to identify, let alone deal with, problems of illiteracy or semi-literacy.'

In 1986, with the support of the Educational and Benevolent Trust, Jill Hutchings produced a report entitled *Dyslexia, Crime and the Probation Service.* A survey of London probation officers revealed that while all were conscious of the literacy problems of their clients, very few linked these to dyslexia. Only one had had any training in dyslexia.

As part of her research Jill Hutchings interviewed a number of prisoners who had been tested for dyslexia. One, Toni, aged thirty-two, who was serving a sentence for theft, she described in the following terms:

> Toni comes from a middle-class family and his father is a professor of history. Despite such a background Toni failed to attain qualifications at school and always had serious difficulties in reading and writing. Toni was referred to the Learning Difficulties Support Service of the Inner London Education Authority by his probation officer and was diagnosed as dyslexic at the age of thirty-one. He felt relieved by the diagnosis of the problem and now feels altogether more confident about his handicap, although he wishes he had been diagnosed earlier.

Spurred on by such examples Jill Hutchings became involved in wider research, for a BBC television programme, to try to assess the extent of dyslexia amongst the inmates of prisons. The result was the BBC 'Public Eye' documentary, broadcast in June 1992. This produced some startling figures, indicating that more than 50 per cent of prisoners could be dyslexic.

The researchers undertook the Bangor Dyslexia Test with 116 randomly selected prisoners and ex-offenders in a number of centres, including Pentonville and Belmarsh prisons, bail hostels in London and amongst ex-offenders' groups in Manchester. The Bangor Test, devised by Professor Tim Miles and detailed in his book *Dyslexia: The Pattern of Difficulties*, is scored on a scale from 0 to 10. In the appropriate context any score of 5 or more is usually taken as positive evidence for dyslexia. Of the 116 tested by the 'Public Eye' researchers, fifty-five had scores of 4 or less (with only two scoring 0), and sixty-one had scores between 5 and 10 – that is, 52 per cent of the sample.

The researchers commented:

> With experience of testing, one gets a gut feeling as to the point at which dyslexia is clearly a handicap for the person being tested. We found that to be about 4 or 5 on the Bangor Test scale. Some who scored 4 seemed to have very clear signs of dyslexia, while others we were less sure about. We therefore made 5 our cut-off point, so as to err on the side of certainty. It's worth noting that there were a very high number of 4s.

In her 1986 study, Jill Hutchings concluded:

> Whilst it is important to stress that there were a number of other problems as well as literacy with all the clients interviewed – for example, drug abuse, severe emotional disturbances, and unemployment – it nonetheless is clear from this small sample of clients that a dislike of school often enhanced by an inability to master reading and writing which resulted in truanting and an inability to find employment, led to subsequent offending.

She said that the prisoner she interviewed, Toni, summarized the relationship most succinctly when he told her: 'I think because people can't read and write they are labelled as an outcast in society and then they commit crime.'

'YOU'LL NEVER AMOUNT TO MUCH'

On the mantelpiece of the Spiers family profiled in Chapter 4 stands a figure of this century's most famous scientist, possibly the most famous of all time, Albert Einstein (1879–1955). His lifelike representation is placed there to remind the family that while, for the most part, dyslexia is a hidden handicap, it is a condition that can also have hidden advantages.

Einstein, of course, along with a phalanx of other luminaries, from Leonardo da Vinci, Auguste Rodin, Gustave Flaubert, Lewis Carroll and Hans Christian Andersen to Charles Darwin, Franklin Roosevelt, Winston Churchill and William Butler Yeats, is believed to have been dyslexic. It is a controversial assertion since the historical evidence is a matter of interpretation. None the less these people's experiences are worth taking into account for what they tell us about different ways of perceiving and interpreting the world.

In his study, *In the Mind's Eye*, the American writer Thomas G. West explores the way creative genius has been allied to thinking in terms of images rather than words or numbers. All the famous personalities listed above appear to have this in common. According to West, new developments in computer technology herald a significant shift towards the increased use of visual approaches to information analysis. As he puts it, 'New opportunities are currently unfolding that may require special talents and abilities in just those areas where many individuals with learning difficulties often have their greatest strengths.'

The opportunities West is talking about include the visualization of scientific concepts and the analysis and manipulation of complex, three-dimensional information, graphically displayed on personal computers. As he says:

> In the future we might see the solution of difficult problems in statistics, molecular biology, materials development, or higher mathematics coming from people who are graphic artists, sculptors, craftsmen, film-makers, or designers of animated computer graphics. Different kinds of problems and different kinds of tools may require different talents and favour different kinds of brains.

Albert Einstein seems to have been a very good early example of this general point. He did not talk until he was three years old, and there was much concern about his development within the family. For example, his sister Maja Wintelere-Einstein recorded: 'He had such difficulty with language that those around him feared he would never learn to speak. . . . Every sentence he uttered, no matter how routine, he repeated to himself, softly moving his lips. This habit persisted until his seventh year.'

There were many examples of frustration in his early education. For instance, when he was five he had a special tutor for lessons and music but had such a tantrum on one occasion, throwing a chair at his teacher, that she left and never returned. At about this time Einstein's father showed him a magnetic compass. He became fascinated with the object, enquiring into the mechanisms which maintained its static position. He himself reported this as having become almost an obsession which directed his thinking for many years afterwards. It was quite evident, before he was ten, that he was unusually skilful in the manipulation of spatial objects – geometric puzzles in particular, and even such complicated ones as the Pythagorean theorem. At the age of twelve he was given a geometry book which still survives, marked and annotated, and which Einstein considered to have played a crucial part in his intellectual development.

However, in formal terms he was regarded as a mediocre student. His sister records that when he entered primary school, aged seven, he had

> a rather strict teacher whose methods included teaching children arithmetic and especially the multiplication tables, with the help of whacks on the hands, so-called 'Tatzen' (knuckle raps); a style of teaching that was not unusual at the time, and that prepared the children early for their future role as citizens.
>
> The boy, self-assured and thorough in thought, was considered only moderately talented, precisely because he needed time to mull things over and didn't respond immediately with the reflex answer desired by the teacher. Nothing of his special aptitude for mathematics was noticeable at the time; he wasn't even good at arithmetic in the sense of being quick and accurate, though he was reliable and persevering. Also, he always confidently found the way to solve difficult word problems, though he easily made errors in calculation.

So, in the area of speed and accuracy of calculation and response – still widely considered to be the main early indicator of mathematical aptitude – Einstein was not especially bright. There is strong evidence, too, that, as he put it himself, he had a 'poor memory for words'. This was doubtless linked to his poor performance with foreign languages, a weakness that stayed with him throughout his life. In 1923, when he was in his mid-forties, he visited Palestine. Despite his new-found enthusiasm for Zionism, he declared that there was little point in his studying Hebrew. According to the diary of one of the officials who received him shortly after his arrival in Palestine, Einstein made 'a little speech explaining the nature of his brain which he said was such that he was afraid it would be unproductive work for him to attempt to learn Hebrew'.

However, where Einstein showed promise was in the area of mathematical intuition associated with spatial imagination. When he was fifteen the family moved from Germany to Italy so that Einstein's father could start a new business near Milan. The intention was for Albert to stay in Munich to finish his schooling, but his dislike of school was so intense that he became, according to one biographer, a drop-out. In a letter he wrote later in life he recalled that his teacher had accused him of creating disruption in the class adding, in the oft-quoted statement, 'You will never amount to much.'

Einstein said that naturally he wanted to follow his family to Milan, but the main reason for his wanting to leave the Munich *Gymnasium* was 'the dull, mechanized method of teaching. Because of my poor memory for words, this presented me with great difficulties that it seemed senseless for me to overcome them. I preferred, therefore, to endure all sorts of punishments rather than learn to gabble by rote.'

Not long afterwards, however, Einstein was fortunate to be able to attend a small progressive cantonal school at Aarau in Switzerland. This placed special emphasis on individual development, relying on visual methods of study. Within the school there was a minimum of verbal communication and a maximum use of diagrams, charts, maps and demonstrations. While there, at the age of sixteen, Einstein wrote his first known scientific paper, entitled 'Concerning the investigation of the state of ether in magnetic fields'.

Einstein graduated from the Zurich Polytechnic in 1900, but remained out of work for more than a year. He tried unsuccessfully to get a teaching job, and gave private lessons for three francs an hour. He lived frugally, ate so little that his health suffered, and became profoundly depressed. Eventually he found a part-time tutoring job, followed by a lowly position as a junior clerk in the Swiss Patent Office. It was some years before his publications won him the career and recognition he deserved.

Reviewing Einstein's early education Thomas G. West remarks on the paradox which it reveals of brilliance combined with examination failure. His difficulties, he says, should not be glossed over and simply explained away in terms of unrecognized genius:

> One of the more distinctive and frightening elements of the experience shared by those with dyslexia and other forms of learning difficulties is the intensification of the crisis period experienced by many in late adolescence and early adulthood. This critical time is

difficult for many without special learning problems, but it can be more so for those we are considering.

Especially when there is no overt recognition of the paradoxical pattern of high talents and substantial disabilities, the sufferer is confronted with internal and external conflict along with confusion along all sides . . . As they approach the responsibilities of adulthood, the highly gifted with learning problems see that their time is running out. Their education is coming to an end, but they see their dreams and prospects fading before their eyes. They have failed examinations or barely passed them.

They are confused by the clarity of their own perceptions and the disapproval of their professors, parents and peers. They may have glimpsed the heights but their confidence has been shaken repeatedly. Their academic record is mixed, at best their references lukewarm. Their fierce honesty and impatience with conventional views, coupled with lack of tact and social grace, may have caused them to make enemies they can ill afford to have. Employment prospects are not good. The dark clouds of depression descend. How many are lost at this stage, we might well wonder.

As it was, in Einstein's case within a few years of this period he went on to make his most creative interventions. In 1905, when he was only twenty-six years old, he published five papers on entirely different subjects, three of them among the greatest in the history of physics. One, of course, was his special theory of relativity in which he amalgamated space, time and matter into one fundamental unity. As C. P. Snow, the physicist and novelist, observed:

This last paper contains no references and quotes no authority. All of the papers are written in a style unlike any other theoretical physicist's. They contain very little mathematics. There is a good deal of verbal commentary. The conclusions, the bizarre conclusions, emerge as though with the greatest of ease: the reasoning is unbreakable. It looks as though he had reached the conclusions by pure thought unaided, without listening to the opinions of others. To a surprisingly large extent, that is precisely what he had done.

Describing these thought processes much later, in 1945, Einstein recorded the following reflections:

The words or the language, as they are written or spoken, do not seem to play any role in my mechanism of thought. The psychical entities which seem to serve as elements in thought are certain signs and more or less clear images which can be voluntarily reproduced and combined.

There is, of course, a certain connection between those elements and relevant logical concepts. It is also clear that the desire to arrive finally at logically connected concepts is the emotional basis of this rather vague play with the above mentioned elements. But taken from a psychological standpoint, this combinatory play seems to be the essential feature in productive thought – before there is any connection with logical construction in words or other kinds of signs which can be communicated to others.

The above mentioned elements are, in my case, of visual and some of muscular type. Conventional words or other signs have to be sought for laboriously only in a secondary stage, when the mentioned associative play is sufficiently established and can be reproduced at will.

Without having the benefit of today's accumulated mass of research and publications on dyslexia, Einstein was here describing how the dyslexic-conditioned mind can function in a creatively original way. Commenting on the passage, Thomas G. West remarks:

It is of no small significance that Einstein's words clearly describe a two-mode process that corresponds closely to the findings of those who have been investigating the roles of the two hemispheres of the brain.

He first *plays* with *images* in the visual right hemisphere, the apparent source of new ideas or perceptions of order, possibly relatively independently of conventional thought, current scientific understanding and education. He plays until he arrives at the desired result. And then, *only in a secondary stage*, does he have to seek *laboriously* for the right words and mathematical symbols to express the ideas in terms of the verbal left hemisphere, in terms of the world, in terms that fit within the structure of scientific thinking, in terms that can be *communicated to others*.

And as one of Einstein's biographers, Gerald Holton, put it in his essay, 'On trying to understand scientific genius':

It is coming to be more widely agreed that an apparent defect in a particular person may merely indicate an imbalance in our normal expectations. A noted deficiency should alert us to look for a proficiency of a different kind in the exceptional person. The late usage of language in childhood, the difficulty learning foreign languages . . . may indicate a polarization or displacement in some of the skill from the verbal to another area. That other, enhanced area is without doubt, in Einstein's case, an extraordinary kind of visual imagery that penetrates his very thought processes.

This is a judgement that can be made about very many dyslexic people, regardless of their general ability measured in terms of intelligence. The key element, always, is recognition, understanding, support and encouragement. In Einstein's case it is likely that the critical period was the time he spent when he was fifteen and sixteen at the small Swiss cantonal school. There, perhaps unknowingly, an entirely appropriate teaching formula was applied to him. As the American neurologist Richard Masland commented:

> It appears that Einstein's development was made possible only by a series of fortuitous almost trivial circumstances, occurring primarily outside of the framework of his formal education. How fortunate that his environment made this possible.
>
> But to maintain a true perspective in this fascinating history, we must not forget its unsung hero – someone must have taught him to read.

'A GOOD LISTENING TO'

We live in a world where success, however it is measured, demands literacy. Moreover, all too often success is also ti'd together with academic attainment. At a very minimum, to survive an adult must be able to negotiate what can be labyrinthine complexities of forms, tax returns, mortgages and the rest. Not to be able to cope with such basic requirements can mean remaining on the sidelines of society.

Exclusion can begin with a person's earliest days at school, as many of the experiences related in this book amply testify. In adulthood it can lead to dyslexics developing elaborate stratagems to fool neighbours and relatives, a kind of espionage of everyday living. In Britain it is estimated that more than two million people are functionally illiterate, many of them as a result of dyslexia.

Part of the problem is the very emphasis placed by society on literacy and related academic achievement. No one would deny the desirability of basic literacy. Yet academic qualifications are no guarantee of success, let alone happiness. In early 1993 a Ciba Foundation conference of psychologists, educationalists, neurobiologists and geneticists from around the world met in London to examine the origins and development of high ability. They agreed that the talents of thousands of young people were being wasted because educational systems measured academic success rather than practical, creative or interpersonal skills.

Professor Robert Sternberg, of Yale University, has made a study of high-achieving academic students and how their careers develop in later life. He told the conference that apart from predicting university results, school examination scores had no correlation with later success. They were of no use, he said, in predicting research ability, teaching ability, creativity or practical abilities, and were only weakly linked to analytic skills:

> Many people with high test scores at school will get good university grades. But this doesn't indicate they will be successful in later life, while people with lower scores may be more successful. The bottom line is that we need to recognize and think about giftedness in ways other than just looking at academic standards. What matters at school doesn't matter nearly so much in later life.

Practical intelligence, Professor Sternberg continued, was of much more use than academic intelligence. *Tacit knowledge* – the ability to learn how to succeed at work – would bring greater success. 'It's the tricks of the trade you learn on the job which are important,' Professor Sternberg said.

> Tacit knowledge is not correlated with IQ. Academic tests do not predict this.
> We need to change the measures we use to look for practical intelligence, not just academic abilities. Many people at the top, the entrepreneurs and captains of industry who are successful, have not been straight A students. We should provide environments which encourage, not discourage, these attributes.
> Parents should look at what their children like and what they are good at and encourage them in this, not have preconceived ideas that they should be a violinist, say, or a doctor.

All of this is especially sound advice for parents of dyslexic children. It is sound advice, too, for schools and teachers. The lives of many thousands of dyslexic children could be made infinitely more tolerable if there was greater understanding of and accommodation for their particular needs and difficulties in often quite small ways. An instance from the school life of Tomos, whose story opened the pages of this book, makes the point. Early on in his secondary school, and in common with very many dyslexic children, Tomos found French lessons particularly onerous. On investigation it transpired that a major part of the problem was copying from the blackboard. Copying is a well-trodden minefield for probably a large majority of dyslexic children. By the time they've looked down at their book they can all too easily have forgotten what they looked up at a moment before. Tomos said the problem was magnified twice over when he was looking up at totally unfamiliar words in another language. The result was that he was being left further and further behind, becoming more and more anxious, and in danger of giving up on the subject altogether. The whole family grew to learn when a day was looming that contained a French lesson.

A solution was found after several conversations with teachers at the school. Tomos simply moved class to learn French from a teacher who made more use of conversational methods, rather than the more traditional blackboard approach.

The problem for the schools, however, is that more and more they are being forced through the requirements of the National Curriculum to a rigid, inflexible approach. More often than not the only answer is in the hands of the parents who, if they deploy patient insistence, can usually negotiate an accommodation. In most cases schools and teachers are only too anxious to ease the path. The problem is generally with the Department for Education insisting on centralized and rigid 'syllabuses', 'standards' and 'tests'.

In 1978 a government inquiry chaired by Baroness Warnock led directly to the 1981 Education Act which specified in a radical way how children with special needs should be treated. Local education authorities were required to draw up Statements assessing the needs of children with physical and mental disabilities or learning difficulties. Yet in early 1993 Baroness Warnock said that the special educational needs of an estimated one million children – that is, one in five and including many with dyslexia – were not being met because local education authorities were failing to assess their learning difficulties.

Where Statements are made they often take an intolerably long time to materialize, as many parents of dyslexic children will testify. In 1992 an Audit Commission report found that some pupils were having to wait for up to three years for a Statement of Special Needs, and the average wait was twelve months. Government guidelines say that children should be assessed within six months.

It is clear what should be done. Schools and teachers should be made much more aware of the children in their care with special needs, including those with dyslexia. Special needs, and especially dyslexia, should be an important part of the training of all teachers, and not just those specializing in remedial work. There should be regular and automatic screening for dyslexia of all children who display literacy and development problems at a young age, around six or seven. Dyslexic children can be recognized by teachers who have had relatively little extra training. When appropriate educational strategies are undertaken and carried out conscientiously, such children need not lead lives of fear and failure.

Of course, such an effort would entail costs and an inconvenience to the system as presently operated. But the costs of not making these changes are incalculable. The costs are those children who fail, who become disruptive, who are effectively excluded from school altogether, and who are pushed along the road to delinquency and crime.

As for parents, a simple message is not to become over-anxious about academic achievement. Anxiety itself is often the fundamental problem for dyslexics, intimately connected with low self-esteem. Research has found, for instance, that normally achieving adolescents tend to attribute their success to their own abilities, and failures to outside causes. Dyslexic adolescents, on the other hand, tend to identify any success with the extent to which they have worked extremely hard, and failure to their own lack of ability.

Dyslexia should rather be seen as an extraordinary dimension of otherwise ordinary life. It has an undeniable downside in terms of the extra effort invariably required, but a positive aspect as well in terms of creative ability. Above all, dyslexic children more than others should not be rushed through their childhood. What they need, as one wise teacher once put it, is 'a good listening to'. And as another declared: 'Children have but *one* childhood. It should not be wasted.'

Appendix

Recognizing Dyslexia

If the answer to three or four of the following questions is *yes* it is quite possible that the person concerned is dyslexic to some extent:

If s/he is aged about eight or under

- Is s/he having particular difficulty with reading or spelling? Does this surprise you? Do you get the impression that in matters not connected with reading and spelling s/he is alert and bright?
- Does s/he put letters the wrong way round, for instance b and d? Does s/he put figures the wrong way round, for example 15 for 51 or 2 for 5? In calculations does s/he need to use bricks or his/her fingers or marks on paper to help?
- Does s/he have unusual difficulty in remembering arithmetical tables?
- Was s/he late in speaking? Does s/he have difficulty in telling left from right?
- Is s/he unusually clumsy? Some dyslexic children show clumsiness, but by no means all. Does s/he find kicking/catching a ball difficult? Do shoelaces/ties, changing/dressing present problems?

If s/he is aged eight to twelve

- Does s/he still make apparently 'careless' mistakes in reading? Does s/he still make strange spelling mistakes? Does s/he sometimes leave letters out of a word? Does s/he sometimes put letters in the wrong order?
- Does s/he have a poor sense of direction and is still sometimes confused over left and right? Are there still occasional b–d confusions? Does s/he still find arithmetical tables difficult?

- Does s/he take much longer than average to do written work at school and at home? Does reading comprehension seem slower than expected for his or her age and intelligence? Does s/he have difficulty in copying from the blackboard at school? Does s/he typically miss out words or a line altogether, or when reading aloud read the same line twice? Does s/he dislike reading aloud?
- Does s/he do much reading for pleasure? Does s/he lack self-confidence and have a poor opinion of himself or herself?

It follows that there are some basic and very simple 'dos' and 'don'ts' advice for parents and teachers in dealing with dyslexic children:

Don't simply brand him or her as lazy or careless.
Don't make invidious comparisons with others in the family or with others in the class at school.
Don't exert undue pressure.
Don't expect him or her to read aloud to others.
Don't be surprised if s/he becomes easily tired and/or discouraged.
Don't be surprised if his or her handwriting is untidy and irregular.
Don't be surprised by inconsistencies, performing well on some occasions and less well on others, often at the same task.

Do encourage him or her in the things s/he does well.
Do read aloud to him or her as often as possible.
Do discuss frankly the things that s/he finds difficult.
Do praise effort and help him or her to recognize that there are plenty of things s/he can do well.

Resource Guide

ORGANIZATIONS: NATIONAL CENTRES

The British Dyslexia Association

98 London Road
Reading RG9 5AU
Tel. (0734) 668271

A charity that co-ordinates a widespread network of local associations and support groups throughout England. It offers support and information to children, adults and professionals, and runs a full advisory service on all aspects of education and training. For an information pack send a large SAE with (currently) a 36p stamp.

Scotland

Scottish Dyslexia Association
Cakemuir House
Nenthorn
Kelso
Roxburghshire TD5 7RY
Tel. (0753) 24806

The Dyslexia Institute (Scotland)
74 Victoria Crescent Road
Dowanhill
Glasgow G11 9JN
Tel. (041) 334 4549

Wales

South Wales Dyslexia Association
4 Dinas Road
Penarn
South Glamorgan CF64 3PL
Tel. (0222) 703124

Dyslexia Unit
University College of North Wales
Bangor
Gwynedd LL57 2DG
Tel. (0248) 351151 Ext. 2203

Northern Ireland

The Northern Ireland Dyslexia Association
7 Mount Pleasant
Stranmilis Road
Belfast BT9 5DS

Republic of Ireland

Dyslexia Association of Ireland
31 Stillorgan Park
Black Rock
County Dublin

USA

The Orton Dyslexia Society
724 York Road
Baltimore
Maryland 21204

Canada

Association of Children and Adults with Learning Disabilities
Maison Kildare House
323 Chapel Street
Suite 200
Ottawa K1N 7Z2

Australia

SPELD
PO Box 94
Mosman 2088
New South Wales

New Zealand

SPELD
PO Box 13391
Christchurch

SPECIALIST ORGANIZATIONS

The Dyslexia Institute

133 Gresham Road
Staines
Middlesex TW18 2AJ
Tel. (0784) 463851

Provides advice, private assessments, teaching and training courses in a
UK network of centres. Fees available on request (bursaries available for
those on low incomes).

Watford Dyslexia Institute

47 Little Oxhey Lane
South Oxhey
Watford WD1 5HN
Tel. 081–421 4266

Provides information, tuition (preferably in schools), assessments and
training. Operates a flexible payment policy.

The Dyslexia Teaching Centre

23 Kensington Square
London W8 5HN
Tel. 071–937 2408

Offers courses, conferences, assessments and one-to-one tuition.

Helen Arkell Centre

Frensham
Farnham
Surrey GU10 3BW
Tel. (025125) 2400/4446

Provides information, counselling, tuition and training.

Hornsby Centre

71 Wandsworth Common West Side
London SW18 2ED
Tel. 071-871 2846

Offers advice, counselling and teaching.

Advisory Centre for Education (ACE)

1b Aberdeen Studios
22-4 Highbury Grove
London N5 2EA
Helpline: Tel. 071-354 8321 - open weekdays 2-5 pm

During the process of 'Statementing' ACE can advise parents where they stand legally - in particular, the respective roles and powers of the headteacher, school governors, the LEA and central government. It can also help parents to find effective ways of making representations about educational issues that may be troubling them. Publishes *The Special Education Handbook*, 5th edn (price £4.50 inc. p&p).

Parents in Partnership

Top Portakabin
Clare House
St George's Hospital
Blackshaw Road
London SW17 0QT
Tel. 081-767 3211

Provides advice on all kinds of special needs.

THE CHANNEL 4 'DYSLEXIA' VIDEO
Produced by Poseidon Film Productions

This is the video of the Channel 4 programme researched by John Osmond, which inspired his book *The Reality of Dyslexia*. It features eight children and adults of different ages – several of whom are described in the book.

Shows the relief diagnosis brings, the importance of early recognition and the tragic consequences of undiagnosed dyslexia. It offers a message of hope and help.
British Dyslexia Association

An excellently produced video that portrays the perception of a range of dyslexics and their families for any audience. It will increase awareness and give invaluable insight into the discovery, assessment, teaching of and living with dyslexia.
Helen Arkell Dyslexia Centre

The key, it is emphasised, is early diagnosis – and teachers trained to recognise the signs of dyslexia. This programme, much acclaimed when it was shown, could go a long way to helping teachers recognise signs, and alert them to the misery dyslexia can cause. It would be difficult to watch it and remain unmoved.
Times Educational Supplement

This video would provide a very valuable resource for all schools in alerting teachers to the symptoms of dyslexia.
National Association of Headteachers' Bulletin

Staff Development Officers in schools could do worse than devoting a day to raising staff awareness through this video.
The Teacher

All teacher training colleges should see this video. This applies to all European teacher training colleges. As this video demonstrates, more than words can state, a dyslexic person's happiness and ultimate achievements will depend so much on early diagnosis of this specific learning difficulty.
Robin Slater, President, European Dyslexia Association

This video manages to pack a tremendous amount into 50 minutes. It succeeds admirably in portraying the reality of dyslexia. It shows the difficulties and the 'normality' of dyslexic individuals, and provides reliable information about causes and the appropriate kinds of help. It would be an excellent focus for professional discussion and in-service training.
Ann Cooke, Dyslexia Unit, University of Wales

All teacher training students should see this video and be given guidance on how dyslexia can be recognised and to whom to go for help.
British Dyslexia Association *Contact* Magazine

The Channel 4 'Dyslexia' Video   Viewing Time: 52 mins   Price: £16.95 (inc. P&P)

TO ORDER

Please send a cheque for £16.95 payable to Hopeline Videos at:
PO Box 515, London SW15 6LQ
(with your name, address, phone number and video title).

Reading List

Augur, J. (1988) *This Book Doesn't Make Sens, Cens, Sns, Scens, Sense: Living and Learning with Dyslexia*. Bath: Bath Educational Publishers.

Augur, J. and Briggs, S. (1992) *The Hickey Multi-sensory Language Course*. London: Whurr, 2nd edn.

British Dyslexia Association (n.d.) *Dyslexia: Your Questions Answered*. Reading: British Dyslexia Association.

Chasty, H. and Friel, J. (1993) *Caught in the Act: Children with Special Needs*. London: Jessica Kingsley, 2nd edn.

Hampshire, S. (1981) *Susan's Story*. London: Sidgwick & Jackson.

Hampshire, S. (1991) *Every Letter Counts: Winning in Life despite Dyslexia*. London: Corgi, 2nd edn.

Hornsby, B. (1988) *Overcoming Dyslexia*. London: Macdonald Optima, 2nd edn.

Innes, P. (1991) *Defeating Dyslexia – A Boy's Story*. London: Kyle Cathie.

Miles, T. R. (1990) *Understanding Dyslexia*. Bath: Amethyst Books (5 West Ave, Oldfield Park, Bath BA2 3QE).

Miles, T. R. (1993) *Dyslexia: The Pattern of Difficulties*. London: Whurr, new edition.

Miles, T. R. and Miles, E. (1990) *Dyslexia a Hundred Years On*. Milton Keynes: Open University Press.

Ostler, C. (1991) *Dyslexia: A Parents' Survival Guide*. Godalming: Ammonite Books (58 Coopers Rise, Godalming, Surrey GU7 2NJ).

Pumfrey, P. D. and Reason, R. (1991) *Specific Learning Difficulties (Dyslexia): Challenges and Responses*. London: Routledge.

Ryden, M. (1992) *Dyslexia: How Would I Cope?* London: Jessica Kingsley, 2nd edn.

West, T. G. (1991) *In the Mind's Eye: Visual Thinkers, Gifted People with Learning Difficulties, Computer Images, and the Ironies of Creativity*. Loughton, Essex: Prometheus (available from Lavis Marketing, 73 Lime Walk, Headington, Oxford OX3 7AD).

Index